FOOD
ADDICTION
DENIAL

False Information and Irrational Thinking

PHILIP WERDELL, M.A.

Philip Werdell, M.A., author of this book, has worked professionally with over 5,000 late-stage food addicts. He is the founder of ACORN Food Dependency Recovery Services and the Food Addiction Institute.

ISBN 978-1-66785-352-9 eBook 978-1-66785-353-6

This book is dedicated to
Carl and Cassie Segal
for their decades-long support
of the Food Addiction Institute
and of this writing.

Contents

Postscript

Why Food Addiction Denial?

Denial is a major characteristic of addiction, and it is certainly a key problem when it comes to chemical dependency on sugar and other hyper-processed foods. Denial is an issue of consciousness. A major aspect of food addiction is that those who have it do not think they have it, and those who are treating it professionally do not think that it is a serious problem.

There are three levels of food addiction denial: 1) cognitive denial, which is when facts are inaccurate and reasoning is incorrect; 2) biochemical denial, where addictive foods, e.g., sugar, flour, caffeine, etc., create physical craving, mental obsession, and an addictive personality; 3) social or institutional denial, where people with power in institutions central to our society's food supply hurt consumers (sometimes intentionally, sometimes unintentionally), then come up with arguments to normalize these practices and build them into the woodwork such that the very fabric of society becomes toxic.

This book starts at the beginning and is primarily about cognitive food addiction denial. Biochemical and institutional food addiction denial are summarized in Appendices A and B.

Food addiction begins with physical craving. Physical craving distorts the hunger instinct for some people, making these people want more food than they need. This physical craving is a biochemical brain change caused by extra sugar or other hyper-processed foods. When this craving happens, food addicts experience a slow but steady increase in their attraction to the trigger food. So, for example, initial overeating of a little extra sugar over time creates an even stronger yearning for more sugar.

During this process, the brain sometimes develops compulsive thoughts that both anticipate the desire for more sugar and set up the conditions for even stronger physical cravings. These thoughts become obsessive and override normal cautionary warnings that remind a person that overeating leads to gaining weight—an undesired result.

Thus, cravings progressively lead to mental distortions. Mental distortions create a pattern of slow but steadily worsening overeating. All this happens at an unconscious level. "Food addicts" seldom realize any change in their thinking has occurred but wonder why they can't control their eating. It doesn't even occur to them that they might be addicted to certain trigger foods that cause them to overeat. *They are in food addiction denial.* Similarly, health professionals working with those who are food addicted often do not recognize that this brain change is key to the obesity they are trying to treat, as well as to other resulting secondary diseases caused by the obesity. *These professionals are also in food addiction denial.*

So why is food addiction denial important? Because a large percentage of those who are overweight or obese, as well as those with diabetes, heart disease, and some cancers, cannot be accurately diagnosed or effectively treated without attending to the issue of food addiction denial.

During my many years as a professional working with food addicts, I developed a fairly long list of reasons people gave for not being food addicted. Some they learned from professionals they had gone to previously for help.

This book addresses several myths—incorrect facts and irrational thoughts about food addiction. If it sparks your interest, read on!

Ten Common Statements Of Food Addiction Denial

Denial Statement #1: Food addiction is not real: There is no scientific evidence establishing food as an addiction.

Denial Statement #2: Food addiction cannot be treated like other addictions: You cannot stop eating completely.

Denial Statement #3: If the problem is eating specific foods, then stop eating them or eat less.

Denial Statement #4: Sugar is natural, and the body needs sugar for energy. Eliminating sugar completely to treat food addiction is unhealthy.

Denial Statement #5: Some people are able to lose weight and maintain it by diet and exercise; others should be able to do this also.

Denial Statement #6: If someone has lost control over their eating, they should go to a therapist or eating disorder specialist to resolve "underlying issues."

Denial Statement #7: There is no evidence that food addiction can be treated effectively.

Denial Statement #8: No one ever robbed a bank to buy sugar or junk food; the personal and social consequences for food addiction are not as serious as they are for alcoholism or other drug addictions.

Denial Statement #9: Bariatric surgery is the only effective treatment for obesity.

Denial Statement #10: No one forces obese people to overeat; obviously, they are the ones who put the food in their mouths. Focusing on personal powerlessness over food is counterproductive; it brings a person down rather than building up self-esteem.

FOOD ADDICTION DENIAL
NO. 1

<u>Denial Statement #1</u>: "Food addiction is not real: there is no scientific evidence establishing food as an addiction."

<u>Rebuttal:</u> Tens of thousands of self-assessed—and often medically diagnosed—food addicts are keeping their disease in remission by treating themselves with an abstinence-abased model,[1] and the scientific evidence for food addiction is overwhelming.[2]

CHAPTER 1

THE SCIENCE OF FOOD ADDICTION

Medicine is a very pragmatic science. If the prescribed treatment for a disease works, that is evidence that the diagnosis is correct.

The initial research establishing food as an addiction is quite substantial. Uncounted early-stage food addicts couldn't stop overeating until they eliminated added sugar and other binge food(s) completely.[3] Since 1960, tens of thousands of middle-stage food addicts who could not achieve and maintain a healthy weight loss by dieting have gone to Overeaters Anonymous (OA) and five other food-related programs built of the addictive model of abstinence and peer support originated by Alcoholics Anonymous (AA).[4] Almost half have reached an average weight loss of nearly 50 pounds.[5] Thousands of late-stage food addicts for whom diets, eating disorder therapy, and/or Twelve Step participation did not work have been detoxified and treated successfully in professional treatment programs. In outcome surveys, two thirds were abstinent at the time of the research, with half of these maintaining back-to-back food abstinence with Twelve Step aftercare support.[6] The most convincing evidence to possible food addicts is the verbal testimonies of other self-assessed food addicts who have lost excess weight, reduced their cravings, and developed more positive self-esteem when they treated themselves as if they were food addicted. Researchers call this "anecdotal evidence"; but there is more rigorous and systematic research, as indicated below.

Since 1990, several independent lines of scientific research have each established the soundness of a diagnosis of food as a substance use disorder, i.e., food addiction, for some people. These include:

- In-depth interviews of overweight adults unable to diet successfully show all the characteristics of an addiction: physical craving, loss of control, withdrawal, tolerance, progression, fatal, denial and treatable.[7]

- At the Princeton animal research laboratory, mice were put through all the experiments well accepted to test for each characteristic of addiction. They found that animals can be addicted to sugar.[8] This research was replicated and furthered by dozens of other universities and research institutes.[9] This is most convincing to other research scientists.

- At the University of Florida brain research center, CAT scans of overweight adults who lost control of their eating were compared with brain scans of active alcoholics and drug addicts. They were very similar;[10] and again, the studies were replicated.[11] This evidence of food addiction is convincing to physicians and other medical professionals.

- Researchers at UCLA School of Medicine found that many overweight adults—not previously alcoholic or drug addicted—have the same D2 dopamine genetic marker as many alcoholics and drug addicts.[12] This suggests some have a genetic proclivity to food addiction.[13]

- A study at the University of Wisconsin found that Naloxone, an opiate blocker, reduced consumption of high-fat, sweet foods in obese and lean female binge eaters.[14] Naloxone is an ingredient in a new medicine approved for binge eating disorder.[15] About half those diagnosed for binge eating disorder are also positive for food addiction, according to the Yale Food Addiction Assessment Scale.[16]

- Dietetics researchers have regularly found that intermittent excess sugar intake creates endogenous opioids.[17] While the opioid created by digestion of sugar is only mildly addictive, many food addicts eat massive amounts of sugar.[18] This type of endogenous chemical reaction inside the body is different from the chemical change in the brain caused by sugar's passing through in the circulatory system.

- In France, researchers found that sweetness, i.e., sugar or artificial sweeteners, is much more addictive in research animals than cocaine.[19]

- The food industry uses rigorous militarily developed research methods for new foods to find which additives—and in what amounts—create the "bliss point" in consumers.[20]

- Big Food has also found that the addictive pull of one food substance, like sugar, flour, fat or salt, reinforces the chemical dependency of other addictive foods.[21] A massive number of these industrially produced foods are now commonly called "junk foods."

- The good news and the most persuasive case that food addiction is a disease is that when some overeaters are treated as though they are addicted to food substances, the problem goes into remission for a majority of them.[22]

- Key evidence regarding the neurobiology of food addiction that was established between 2001 and 2009 was reconfirmed in new studies in 2013 and 2018.[23]

The major relevant medical associations now accept food as an addiction. The American Society of Addictive Medicine (ASAM) includes food substances as a source of chemical dependency in their evidence-based definition of addiction as a brain disease.[24] The American Psychiatric Association (APA) now asserts that many with eating disorders also show characteristics of food as a substance use disorder.[25] The National Center on Addiction and Substance Abuse (CASA) has a white paper recommending science-based treatment of food addiction. This paper's recommendations suggest the same principles of addiction treatment that are followed in food addiction self-help, food related Twelve Step organizations, and the professional food addiction programs mentioned above.[26]

Dr. Nora Volkow, Director of the National Institute of Drug Abuse at the National Institute of Health, indicated at the 2012 American Psychiatric Association's national conference that there is a consensus among scientists that food addiction is real.

So food addiction is definitely real,[27] and there definitely is a solution.[28]

FOOD ADDICTION DENIAL
NO. 2

<u>Denial Statement #2:</u> "Food addiction cannot be treated like other addictions: You cannot stop eating completely."

<u>Rebuttal:</u> This is a misunderstanding of the treatment language for substance use disorders. "Food abstinence" means completely eliminating the specific food(s) that create physical craving and chemical dependence.

CHAPTER 2

ADDICTIVE FOODS

When alcoholics stop drinking, they do not stop drinking all liquids. They still drink water, tea, coffee, milk, juices, etc. They just refrain completely from drinking alcohol.

When drug addicts stop using drugs, they do not stop using all drugs. They still use aspirin, penicillin, and other medications prescribed by a doctor. They just abstain completely from street and prescription drugs which are addictive.

Similarly, food addicts do not stop eating. They must continue eating a nutritionally balanced diet. They just abstain from their binge foods, the *specific foods* upon which they have become chemically dependent. Dozens of foods have been shown clinically to be addictive, causing cravings and out-of-control eating which were minimized or eliminated when the specific foods were removed completely from the diet.[29] (Note: Some people present as addicted to almost all foods. Such addiction to all foods may be caused by a deficiency of leptin at the cellular level. This is often treated through the practice of "committing to a sponsor" specific amounts of each food and then weighing and measuring.)

What foods can be addictive? The most common addictive food is sugar,[30] followed by flour, fat, artificial sweeteners, and other refined foods.[31] As a part of their food abstinence, a sample of 250 alumni of ACORN Food Dependency Services reported that they completely eliminated entirely different foods:

- Sugar (86% of respondents)

- Volume (74%)

- Alcohol (74%)

- Flour (71%)

- Chocolate (70%)

- At least one other food (44%).[32]

Other specific foods that 44% of respondents eliminated include wheat, artificial sweeteners, caffeine, excess fat, chewing gum, nuts, and salt.

The **addictive potential of sugar and the suggestion of complete abstinence have been well established** in popular books about food addiction:

- Dufty's *Sugar Blues* in 1976,[33]

- Dr. Wunderlich's *Sugar and Your Health* in 1982,[34]

- Hollis's *Fat Is a Family Affair in 1985*,[35]

- Appleton's *Lick the Sugar Habit* in 1996,[36]

- Sheppard's *Food Addiction: The Body Knows*, in 1989,[37]

- Katherine's *Anatomy of a Food Addiction; The Brain Chemistry of Overeating* in 1996,[38]

- Ifland's *Sugars and Flours: How They Make Us Crazy, Sick and Fat and What TO Do About IT* in 1999,[39]

- DesMaisons' *The Sugar Addict's Total Recovery Program* in 2000.[40]

More recently, since an avalanche of scientific research came out about food addiction,[41] several doctors have explained and advocated for the complete elimination of sugar and other specific foods:

- Dr. Lazaro's (with Danowski) *Why Can't I Stop Eating?* in 2009,[42]

- Dr. Bernard's *Breaking the Food Seduction* In 2003,[43]

- Dr. Hyman 's *The Blood Sugar Solution* in 2012,[44]

- Dr. Peeke's *The Hunger Fix* in 2013,[45]

- Dr. Tarman's *Food Junkies: The Truth About Food Addiction* in 2018.[46]

Of course, thousands have been abstaining from sugar in Overeaters Anonymous (OA), back to 1960.[47] Newer addiction-model food-related Twelve Step programs like Food Addicts Anonymous (FAA) in 1987,[48] GreySheeters Anonymous (GSA),[49] and Compulsive Overeaters Anonymous HOW (CEA-HOW)[50] all require food plans with food containing *no added sugar*. (Note: Of course, humans all need sugar on a regular basis in their diets for energy; but there is sufficient sugar nutritionally in fruits and vegetables. The digestive process of these whole foods reduces the amount and the intensity of the sugar in the blood stream.)[51]

What of more subtle and complex situations?

First, these "complexities" often do not arise. Self-assessed food addicts tend to try one of the food plans or definitions of abstinence that they first are convinced might work. For early-stage food addicts trying food abstinence on their own, this might be from a friend or colleague, a mention in the media, a possible sponsor from a free mutual support group, or their personal doctor, dietician, or therapist. Although there is no rigorous research on this subject, my clinical impression after working with over 5000 late-stage food addicts is that **the specific food plan is often not as important as the decision to go to any length to follow it rigorously.**

For example, at Glenbeigh Psychiatric Hospital of Tampa between 1984 and 1996, all clients were asked to follow a single food plan which had a history of working in a Twelve Step context and which was approved by the American Diabetes Association and the American Heart Association. My clinical impression as a therapist there for seven years is that 90% of patients achieved and maintained food abstinence using the prescribed food plan. The dietician modified the plan for the other 10%.[52]

Another example: There is a long history of many members of food-addiction model Twelve Step fellowships—OA-HOW, OA-90 Days, FAA, GSA, FA, CEA-HOW, and RFA—using the food plan suggested or required by each group. Some have their food plan modified by local medical professionals. Many either do not achieve abstinence or drop out. It is unclear whether this is a problem with the food plan's not being appropriate for certain individuals or a problem that individuals do not or cannot surrender to it.[53]

Second, the prescription for sugar addiction abstinence can depend on dosage, timing and context. In early stages, moderate treatments may work, and those whose addiction has reached a critical stage may need to be much more rigorous. Here are common progressive levels of sugar addiction sensitivity:

- No "added sugar," e.g., no sugar in coffee or sprinkled on cereal.
- No "sweets," e.g., such sugary desserts such as ice cream, frosted cake, or candy.
- No sugar in processed foods, e.g., "none up to the 5th ingredient."
- No sugar or "hidden sugars,"[54] e.g., dextrose, barley malt, fructose, honey.
- No sugar, hidden sugars, or artificial sweeteners at all.
- No natural food with high intensity sugar, e.g., dates, ripe bananas, or other tropical fruits.

Just as psychotropic medication is seen as adding a micronutrient to balance brain chemistry, abstinence from a food substance can be understood as subtracting a psychoactive food substance to balance brain chemistry. With medication, this is partly a science and partly an art. There is no serious science about degrees of food abstinence yet; so if a food plan is not working, the decision about what to include in the food plan is almost entirely a trial-and-error experiment.[55]

Third, the brain can become chemically dependent on other specific foods. As the disease progresses, food addicts become addicted to flour[56] and other food substances which have a high glycemic index.[57] Some food addicts need to abstain from wheat, possibly a variant of celiac disease;[58] and others, like Prader-Willi patients, have trouble with volume of all foods, possibly a result of an insufficient amount of the satiety signaling the chemical leptin at the cellular level.[59] Processed foods contain many addictive substances for which no research has been done comparable to the animal studies for sugar addiction.[60]

Some food addicts are genetically predisposed.[61] Others become addicted for environmental reasons: a family where overeating and obesity were highly tolerated, overuse of addictive foods as part of an eating disorder, and increasing amounts of sugar and other addictive foods in the standard American diet. Forty years ago, only minimal processed foods were available in the grocery store, and only 20% contained added sugar. Today, a majority of store foods have been processed, and 80% of these have added sugar.[62]

Fourth, a lot of conflicting information exists about which foods are addictive and which are not. Not all people are food addicted. Just as non-alcoholics can safely drink a variety of alcoholic beverages in moderation, those who are not food addicted can eat all foods in moderation, even overeat at times, and still be able to moderate or stop later.[63] This is evident in the outcome studies of Weight Watchers in which 10-20% are able to achieve and maintain a healthy weight by dieting with support.

However, knowing whether or not you are addicted can be confusing. Early-stage addiction often looks like a normal eater's having periodic binges; middle-stage food addiction often derives from an eating disorder; and late-stage food addiction is usually complicated by other mental and physical diagnoses.[64] Moreover, a food addict's personal health profession-als might have widely varying knowledge and opinions about the disease, many having learned in graduate school, when science was still sparse, that there was no such thing as food addiction.

When newcomers arrive at a support group with other food addicts, they find a wide range of opinions about what is required: What foods do they stop eating? What support do they need? What is suggested regarding the emotional and spiritual dimensions of the disease? Those new to their own abstinence and recovery are often true believers. They think there is only one way, *their* way. Sorting out what to make of this mix of opinions and experience can take time—and trial and error.

There is one certainty: If you *are* food addicted, you can't choose to not be a food addict. Similarly, you cannot choose the food or foods to which you are addicted. In the end, dieting, or just eating moderate meals, will not work for food addicts. Focusing only on underlying psychological issues will not be enough if you are chemically dependent. If nothing else, as they say, the food will teach you.

FOOD ADDICTION DENIAL
NO. 3

<u>Denial Statement #3</u>: "If the problem is eating specific foods, then stop eating them or eat less."

<u>Rebuttal</u>: This is a misunderstanding of addiction; food addicts become powerless over physical cravings, mental obsessions and distortions of will.

CHAPTER 3

THE LIMITS OF REASON

Food addiction, like other substance use disorders, is a brain disease.[65] As the disease progresses, the food addict loses more and more control. First there is physical craving, and food addicts increasingly cannot stop eating their trigger foods once they have started. Second, to counteract attempts to diet and control their food, the disease sets off mental obsessions, during which the food addict believes rationalizations for beginning to eat trigger foods. Third, as cravings and obsessions begin to mingle with neurotic thinking, an addictive personality develops and grows. Each of these biochemical changes hijacks the brain, making it more and more impossible for the addict to stop eating or eat less.

Physical Craving

When the brain of an individual is predisposed, specific foods change the dopamine receptors biochemically such that the brain becomes chemically dependent on the same food that caused the problem. This is physical craving.[66]

Craving is different from hunger. Hunger signals the mind that the body needs nutrition. Craving signals that the mind/body *has* to eat; it is like a *false starving*. Ultimately, individual food addicts experience a sense that it is potentially life-threatening if they don't eat this particular food immediately.[67]

Food addiction is a progressive disease. Each time a craving entices food addicts to eat a particular addictive food, the ingested food changes more dopamine receptors in their brains, and the physical cravings increase. At one point, the food addict becomes powerless over the craving and can no longer resist it. As with alcoholism and other drug addiction, reason and willpower are no longer sufficient to resist.[68] In food addiction, the cravings are generally limited to a few specific trigger foods: added sugar, flour, excess fat, salt, and sometimes too much volume of any food.[69] Unlike with alcoholism or drug addiction, however, in processed foods, these potentially triggering substances are pervasive.[70] The solution is still complete abstinence from processed foods containing trigger substances, such as added sugar.

Abstinence from these specific foods is pretty straightforward, but it does get complicated. The classic AA phrase is that addiction is "subtle, baffling and powerful."[71] For example, it is generally true that a food addict whose disease has reached a critical level cannot stop eating after the first bite of a binge food,[72] but this is not always true. In early addiction, food addicts often still have some control, and this creates a memory that argues that eating the food is safe when it really has become dangerous.[73] Even middle- and late-stage food addicts may seemingly have no trouble overeating some foods for which they have low-level cravings; however, as the eating continues, the disease progresses, and out-of-control eating will return. On the other hand, there are times when just a smell or sight of a trigger food, even just the thought of the food, will spark cravings that cannot be resisted.[74]

A rigorous definition of powerlessness over food craving is: "Food addicts do not know if they will be able to stop eating a trigger food once they start." The solution is complete abstinence from any food that has caused cravings in the past.

Mental Obsession

When cravings have led to negative consequences, e.g., overweight or pre-diabetes, the food addict will resist and try to regain control. At this point, the addictive disease moves beyond the pleasure center and into the cognitive center, the memory center, and the executive center of the brain.[75] This creates impairments in the conscious mind, or mental obsessions.[76] As with alcoholism and drug addiction, the food addict has no defense against this irrational thinking.[77]

Examples of this include: black and white thinking, over generalizing, mental flirting, positive blindness, labeling and mislabeling, personalizing, and minimization.[78] When this is environmentally caused, the irrational thinking can be resolved by rational emotive therapy;[79] however, the biochemically caused irrationality of addiction is more problematic. For example, euphoric recall, mental blackouts, or addictive thinking are often not susceptible to cognitive therapy until after a food addict is abstinent.[80]

If the addictive has blocked out memories of negative consequences (euphoric recall) and selectively all memory (mental black spot), the food addict is powerless over this at the moment it happens. Even when the addict prepares not to be taken in by some irrational argument to overeat, his power to choose is blocked out by the compulsion of addictive thinking.[81]

These are some of the common irrational thoughts food addicts believe: "I feel depressed; the food will make me feel better." "I feel very happy; eating is the best way to celebrate." "The food is free." "Other people are eating it with impunity." "I can't let the food go to waste." "I'm powerless over this food, so I have to eat." "I will start my diet tomorrow." All these and hundreds of other thoughts come up in the addict's mind to rationalize eating when the food addict has previously committed to not eat.[82] Sometimes food addicts are powerless to believe them ... even if they lead to eating a trigger food and being unable to stop.

Lawrie C. calls this "the double whammy":

> The *first part* of our addiction is that we are powerless over food—we get uncontrollable physical craving when we eat certain foods or indulge in certain eating behaviors. This is the **allergy of the body.**

The *second part* is that we cannot manage our lives in relationship to our powerlessness over food—we get obsessions that send us back those foods and those eating behaviors that we know will cause uncontrollable cravings. The is the **obsession of the mind.**

We have what Dr. Silkworth called the "double whammy." We can't stop once we've started; and we can't stop from starting again.[83]

Of course, Lawrie is summarizing the First Step of the Twelve Steps for food addicts. "If Step One is the problem of powerlessness, then Step Two (finding a Power greater than oneself) is the solution."[84] The Twelve Steps are just one of many spiritual paths to experiencing such a power. There are other effective ways to deal with addiction, but this problem presented by Lawrie C and Dr. Silkworth makes a strong case for the food addict's being unable to simply stop eating addictive food(s).

In his book *Addictive Thinking—Understanding Self-Deception,* Dr. Twerski, a psychiatrist and rabbi as well as Director of a noted alcohol and drug rehabilitation center, helps us understand addiction in general, and food addition in particular, as a brain disease with two specific comparisons—first, to dyslexia (p 34) and second, to schizophrenia (pp. 7-8).[85]

Dyslexia helps us understand the physical craving. Both dyslexia and the physical craving are caused by distortions in the brain. Twerski explains dyslexia:

Some people who have this learning disorder "see" letters reversed in words. You ask them to read the word *cat* and they may see TAC or CTA. But they are certain that they have read it accurately. The problem involves their perception of how the letters are organized. The idea does not indicate low intelligence; dyslexia can occur in highly intelligent people.[86]

The physical craving of food addiction mistakes the strong desire for a specific food with natural hunger. Food addicts often unconsciously assume that both sensory stimuli—hunger and craving—are the same

Schizophrenia helps us understand the mental obsessions of food addiction. Twerski explains:

> Therapists familiar with paranoid schizophrenic patients who have delusions of grandeur know how futile it is trying to convince a patient that he or she is not the Messiah or the victim of worldwide conspiracy. The therapist and the patient are operating on completely different wavelengths, with two completely different rules of thought. Normal thinking is absurd to a schizophrenic as schizophrenic thinking is to a healthy person. A typical schizophrenic's adjustment to life in a normal society can be described in terms of a baseball manager who orders his team to punt or a football coach who calls for stealing a base.
>
> Schizophrenic people do not realize that their thinking processes are different from the thinking process of most other people. They can't see why others refuse to recognize them as the Messiah or the victim of a worldwide conspiracy. Still many people, some therapists included, may argue with a schizophrenic person and then become frustrated when the person fails to see the validity of their arguments. This is like asking a color-blind person to distinguish colors.
>
> … Being confronted with the thinking of an alcoholic or someone with another addiction, can be as frustrating as dealing with a schizophrenic.[87]

Both have delusions, hallucinations, inappropriate moods, and very abnormal behavior.

Distortion of Self-Will, or Addictive Personality

As the brain disease of food addiction progresses, memories of crav-ings and active mental obsessions (sometimes integrated with other neu-rotic thinking) form together into a distorted personality.[88] Food addicts believe they are or should be like normal people, but they are also develop-ing a distorted sense of themselves.

In the AA classic *Alcoholics Anonymous*, the alcoholic is described as like Dr. Jekyll and Mr. Hyde, sometimes seeming normal and healthy in every way, and then, suddenly acting quite insane.[89] Similarly, the addictive or diseased part of the brain hijacks the food addict's consciousness; then, when the addict is no longer actively eating or possessed by obsessions, consciousness returns to normal. It is confusing to talk with an active food addict, and even more confusing to be one. "It may be confusing to talk with a schizophrenic, but we are not fooled by a schizophrenic's mind. We are more often taken in by the relative subtlety of the distortions cause by addictive thinking.[90]

As a brain disease, food addiction affects food addicts' consciousness of themselves.

The food addict's problem can be viewed another way. Psychologically, the food addict's powerlessness over food is currently considered a prob-lem of the brain's "executive function," which is the part of the conscious mind that makes decisions and acts on them.[91]

When a distorted hunger instinct becomes unconsciously supported by mental obsession, this addictive thinking begins to distort the food addict's sense of self.[92]

Just as with alcoholism and other drug addictions, the diseased part of the brain hijacks more and more of the food addict's healthy conscious-ness. In late and final stages of food addiction, the distorted thinking forms an addictive personality. Food addicts seldom consider that their physical cravings are not natural hunger. Thus, it also seems logical to assume that their disordered eating is something they are choosing, rather than their being hijacked by their disease. As they are taken in by their own mental obsessions, it is very difficult for them to accept that their experience is importantly different from that of a normal, healthy eater. They constantly struggle to control their food and weight, as other people seem to do so effortlessly. When it is suggested to food addicts that they are powerless over their overeating, they report their experience as, "I am the one who put the food in my mouth."[93]

The disease speaks to food addicts in their own voice. A seamlessness exists between the experience of choosing what clothes to wear and choosing what food to eat, except sometimes food addicts do not follow the commitment to eating that they made to themselves or to others. The fact is that food addicts increasingly lose their power to control their eating; and whether they admit it or not, this is humiliating. "How could I not be able to control what I am eating? This is something any child can do. There must be something wrong with me!"[94]

As the cravings, obsessions, and addictive personality progress, food addicts become increasingly powerless over their own distorted consciousness. They cannot just "put down the food."

Thus, abstaining from addictive foods minimizes or removes cravings, but it leaves in place the more advanced parts of the brain disease—mental obsessions and addictive personality. These two will lead the food addict back into diseased eating.

FOOD ADDICTION DENIAL
NO.4

<u>Denial Statement #4</u>: "Sugar is natural, and the body needs sugar for energy. Eliminating sugar completely to treat food addiction is unhealthy."

<u>Rebuttal:</u> Food addiction treatment for sugar addiction eliminates added sugar. The body continues to obtain the sugar it needs for energy from the natural sugar in a nutritionally balanced diet, and this is healthier than eating progressively more sugar and too many foods that digest into glucose, i.e., the primary form of sugar used by the body for energy. NOTE: Other specific foods must be eliminated if they are triggering a substance use disorder.

CHAPTER 4:

NATURAL SUGAR VS. ADDED PROCESSED SUGAR

Almost all foods break down in part biochemically into glucose sugar. The United Nations World Health Organization (WHO) has recommended that humans need about 8-12 teaspoons of sugar per day to thrive.[95] The sugar in natural products such as fruits and vegetables can account for 6-8 tsp. The average person in the United States ingests about 17 teaspoons of sugar a day, mostly in added processed sugar.[96] Food addicts active in their disease periodically ingest much more sugar than the WHO recommends per day.[97]

Endocrinology

Dr. Robert Lustig, nationally eminent endocrinologist, explains the basic problem: "It is a matter of dosage and timing. When you eat an apple, the sugar enters the blood stream slowly as you digest the roughage. This delay is missing in most processed foods."[98] So when a person eats too much sugar at one time or too high a percentage of highly processed foods, the body gets too much sugar, and it gets it too fast. The insulin mechanism in the body is overloaded, and the excess sugar is stored in fat. Over time, the insulin process speeds up, but it cannot keep up with the progressive increase in dietary sugar. Yet the food addict's addicted brain craves and obsesses for increasingly more dietary sugar.[99]

Brain Chemistry

Parallel to the damage to the endocrine system, increased amounts of sugar flow to the brain through the circulatory system. When there is too much sugar and when there is susceptibility in the brain, the sugar causes biochemical changes in brain receptors. Essentially, the receptors needing sugar to function become weaker and need more frequent and more intense dosages of sugar. This is the science of craving.[100] Sugar and other toxic food substances damage the brain and create a condition in the brain where an increasing amount of sugar is progressively needed to just function "normally."

Different levels of sugar intensity

Unlike alcoholism and other drug addictions, "eliminating sugar completely" is more complex. In recovery practice, food addicts in early stages of the disease often just need to eliminate obvious added sugar, e.g., no sugar in drinks, no sugary desserts.[101] Some food addicts move to one of the many versions of low-carbohydrate diets.[102] By the middle stage of food addiction, most food addicts need to look carefully at the labels of processed foods and remove those with too much added sugar.[103] A common rule in Twelve Step recovery food fellowships is: No sugar up to the first five ingredients on the label.[104] Food addicts at this stage of the disease often also eliminate sugar-intense fruits, e.g., tropical fruits (See Chapter 2). Finally, at the extreme end of this spectrum, some late-stage food addicts find they need to cast aside all fruits and processed foods containing any of the 100 Names for Sugar, as indicated in the Food Addicts Anonymous list.[105]

Foods Other Than Sugar

It is not unusual for food addicts who have eliminated sugar from their diet to find that they are bingeing on grains, particularly highly processed flour. A major reason for this is that the digested sugar from processed grains moves into the bloodstream almost as quickly as processed sugar.[106] Thus, for example, many recovering food addicts in the Twelve Step fellowships begin by eliminating sugar, flour, and alcohol. One of these fellowships, GreySheeters Anonymous, is built around a food plan which eliminates processed grains entirely.[107]

Historically, many food addicts abstaining from sugar have continued to use artificial sweeteners. Unfortunately, some of these folks then became addicted to sugar substitutes. Some people become particularly addicted to excess fat; they need to trim the fat from meat, remove the skin from poultry, minimize the use of sauces and dressings based on anything but a teaspoon of simple olive oil, and eliminate all chocolate.[108] In isolated cases, some food addicts must eliminate all wheat, meat, and cheese.[109]

Most food addicts arrive at the correct "dosage" of sugar and other addictive foods by trial and error. This experimental approach is not as difficult as it might at first seem because, especially in the food-related Twelve Step programs, a great deal of the experimentation has been done by others in the past. For example, almost all those who see themselves as addicted eliminate sweet foods where sugar is a primary ingredient, and almost all who see their addiction as fairly advanced eliminate sugar up to the fifth ingredient in processed foods. Moreover, there is a pattern of selection by observation. It is recommended in OA, for example, that people find others who have a recovery that they want and pattern their eating and recovery practices after that person. Newcomers will often ask such people to be their sponsors. Sponsors will often suggest that newcomers try the food plan that has already worked for the sponsor. When a newcomer does not become abstinent, he or she can change sponsors at will; struggling food addicts will often look for a sponsor who has experienced problems similar to theirs and who has found a food plan that works.

It is important to note that finding the correct food plan is only one task in learning to be abstinent and in recovery from food addiction. Emotional and spiritual problems caused by the disease must also be addressed. A problem for some food addicts is that they keep chasing after the perfect food plan when the real problem might be finding support to surrender to any plan. Practical evidence of this is seen in residential treatment programs where most patients have been unable to be abstinent and all patients are given the same or nearly the same food plan. For example, at the food addiction program of the Glenbeigh Psychiatric Hospital of

Tampa from 1982-1997, all patients were given the same food plan and supported to surrender to this plan rigorously one day at a time.[110] This worked for 90% of the patients; the others needed adjustments in the food plan, either removing further foods or adding snacks or lowering dosages of foods particularly toxic to them.

Problems Caused by the Food Industry

Overeating sugar has long been a problem in the U.S. diet. Older Americans remember the campaigns to "eat less sweets because sugar causes tooth decay."[111] More ominous is the research finding that digested sugar feeds cancer cells, and these cells thrive more in an abundance of sugar than without it.[112] The American Medical Association (AMA) substantiated this finding in 1931 but then rescinded its official caution, but the science has not changed.[113]

Now the problem is more critical, for as sugar has become the predominant addictive food substance, its use continues to rise. Food addiction, like alcoholism and narcotic addiction, is a progressive disease. Sugar addicts keep damaging their brains, and the biochemistry keeps demanding more and more sugar. This is true of other addictive food substances, but we are now just focused on the issue of sugar addiction.

Collectively, sugar addicts keep creating more demand for sugar in all its forms, so now high fructose corn syrup is competing for the market that used to be dominated by cane sugar. This, as well as the advantage of hiding sugar additives under other names the general consumer doesn't recognize, are reasons for the more recent phenomenon, as is stated in the Food Addicts Anonymous pamphlet, "99 Names for Sugar."[114]

As Michael Moss abundantly proves in his best-selling book *Sugar, Salt Fat: How the Food Giants Hooked Us,* the food industry itself has become addicted to adding sugar.[115] Dr. Robert Lustig, Professor of Pediatrics in the Division of Endocrinology at the University of California, San Francisco, where he specializes in neuroendocrinology and childhood obesity, found that 35 years ago, just 20% of processed food sold in grocery stores contained added sugar in some form. Today, not only is significantly more processed food sold, but also, 80% of processed food contains sugar.[116] At a conference of food industry leaders in 1999, it was proposed to start slowly cutting back the amount of sugar in their manufactured foods. One major company, General Mills, said no; and the logic of competition kept all the others from going forward with this constructive proposal.[117] This leaves food addicts—and potential food addicts—with an increasingly dangerous environment in every supermarket and grocery store.

The recent white paper by CASA argues for treating sugar and other addictive food products like we have long treated alcohol and, more recently, successfully treated nicotine. These food products are health hazards, especially to children, and they must be regulated by the government if the food industry continues to be unwilling to self-regulate.[118]

The sugar industry in the United States has always responded to demand and made a substantial profit. Over the last few decades, it has pressed for tariffs on imported sugar. This has raised the price of sugar from other counties and kept domestic sugar prices artificially low.[119] At the same time, sugar lobbyists were successful in selling the public and even the medical establishment that all sugar is "natural"; even that it is a healthy food.[120]

Conclusion: The denial statement that "all sugar is natural and is needed by the body for energy" is a just a subtle and pernicious part of this general problem. Refined sugar is very different from the natural sugar in whole foods. With billions of dollars of advertising money behind it, the amount of added sugar now in the consumer food chain has become a health hazard to the general population and a part of the social denial system about food addiction.

FOOD ADDICTION DENIAL
NO. 5

<u>Denial Statement #5</u>: "Some people are able to lose weight and maintain it by diet and exercise; others should be able to do this also."

<u>Rebuttal</u>: There are people for whom the problem is just weight.[121] We call them Normal Eaters who are overweight or obese. There are other people who have problems of weight who also have eating disorders or food-related substance use disorders.[122] We call them Emotional Eaters with eating disorders and food addicts with a chemical dependency. For Food Addicts who are overweight, the problem is not just weight.

CHAPTER 5

THE LIMITS OF WILLPOWER

Some people *can* lose weight and maintain their weight loss by diet and exercise alone. However, not all overweight and obese people are able to do this because some have an eating order or a food addiction.[123] Obesity, eating disorders, and food addiction are three entirely different diseases. Each requires an entirely different treatment. Sometimes people have two or all three of these diseases, and then all three approaches to treatment are required.

The chart below, "'Normal' Eater, Emotional Eater, Food Addict," outlines the difference between the diseases of obesity, eating disorder, and food chemical dependency, i.e., substance use disorder. The general public and the medical community are frequently confused about these distinctions; thus, they assume all problems of weight are just the disease of obesity. In fact, most food addicts have experienced being overweight or obese, but some have not; and a large percentage of those who have problems with weight also have an eating disorder and/or a food addiction. Thus, the statement "My problem is weight; I am not a food addict" is sometimes true and sometimes a subtle and complex problem of food addiction denial.

"NORMAL" EATER, EMOTIONAL EATER, FOOD ADDICT

"NORMAL" EATER (with obesity)	EMOTIONAL EATER (eating disorder)	FOOD ADDICT (chemical dependency)
The problem is **physical (neuro-hormonal)**: • Weight gain or excess body fat with health complications such as diabetes, sleep apnea, heart disease, arthritis, depression, infertility, liver disease, gout	The problem is **physical and mental-emotional**: • Binge eating, restricting, and/or purging over feelings • Unresolved trauma • And possibly weight (sometimes overweight and sometimes underweight)	The problem is **physical, mental-emotional and spiritual**: • Physical craving (false starving) • Mental obsession (false thinking) • Self-will run riot (false self) • And often trauma and obesity
The solution is **physical (neuro-hormonal)**: • Physician assessment and management of the root causes of weight gain • Physician management of health complications • Improved food choices and eating habits • Physical activity and improved sleep • Support for eating, exercise and lifestyle changes	The solution is **mental-emotional**: • Develop skills to cope with feelings other than with restricting, purging and bingeing • Resolve past emotional trauma and irrational thinking (healing trauma) **... and physical** • And those to the left	The solution is **spiritual**: • Abstinence from binge foods and abusive eating behaviors • Rigorous honesty about all thoughts and feelings • A disciplined spiritual program, e.g., the Twelve Steps or equivalent. **... and mental-emotional and physical** • And all those applicable to the left
What works: • Reason and will power (and sometimes acceptance-based therapy, pharmaceuticals, and bariatric surgery)	What works: • Eating in moderation (along with feeling your feelings)	What works: • Acceptance of your addiction (and all the changes that this implies)

We will begin by describing each of these general categories.

OBESITY

For Normal Eaters who are overweight or even obese, the problem is primarily physical weight. The solution is: "Less calories in and more calories out."[124] Overweight normal eaters need a medically approved diet, an exercise plan, and lifestyle changes which support moderate eating and exercise.

Excellent demographic research exists on obesity worldwide going back several decades.[125]

> According to the Center for Disease Control, the Body Mass Index (BMI) ranges for "underweight," "normal weight," "overweight," "obese," and "extremely obese" are:
>
> If your BMI is less than 18.5, it falls within the underweight range.
>
> If your BMI is 18.5 to <25, it falls within the normal.
>
> If your BMI is 25.0 to <30, it falls within the overweight range.
>
> If your BMI is 30.0 to <40, it falls in the obese range.
>
> If your BMI is 40.0 or higher, it falls in the "extreme" or "severe" obese range.[126]

Currently, two thirds of U.S. adults are overweight; over half of the overweight people are obese; and a small but growing percentage are morbidly obese. According to the Center for Disease Control (CDC), Americans are "the biggest they've ever been, and by far: New government data shows that roughly 100 million people in this country are now **obese**, a "sharp increase" from the previous decade. These numbers—the latest from the National Health and Nutrition Examination Survey [as of March 26, 2018]—put the **rate** of **obese** adults at 39.6%."[127]

In a Consumer Reports survey of 9,000 readers rating 13 diet plans and protocols, the median loss for women over a nine-month period was 15 pounds, and 18 pounds for men. Some adults can have significant weight loss on any of these plans; however, half of those dieting lose less than 16-19 pounds in nine months,[128] and most begin regaining weight after a year.[129]

As with most comparison studies, the Weight Watchers program had the best outcome for commercial programs. Some programs, like Atkins and other low-carb diets, reported larger initial weight loss, but no better results regarding weight loss maintenance. Weight Watchers, now WW, reports a recent six-month clinical trial in which the average weight loss was about 8%. What all of these outcome surveys of weight loss diets show is that some people are able to lose weight by dieting, and some, though fewer, are able to maintain this weight loss. We have described this group as Normal Eaters, i.e., those without eating disorders, food addiction, or other biochemical abnormalities affecting weight.

Case Study: Anthony

When he was about 50 years old, Anthony's doctor became very alarmed by his blood pressure and cholesterol readings and told him that he needed to lose at least 50 pounds and keep it off or he could easily have a heart attack or stroke. Anthony said, "What do I need to do?" The doctor gave him a pre-diabetic exchange diet. He gave it to his wife and said, "Can you please cook this way." When she said *yes,* he also asked her, "How can I eat this way when at work and in restaurants?"

Right there in about an hour, they figured out how he could follow this diet outside the home.

The outcome was that without any problem, Anthony ate this way for the last 25 years of his life. He lost the needed weight in less than a year and never had any interest in returning to his previous way of eating.

My observation is that from that day forward, Anthony had no craving and no food obsession.

Case Study: Marian

One day, Marian came down to breakfast and said she had something really difficult to tell her husband. His first thought was that something had happened to one of the kids. This turned out not to be true. Her problem was, as she put it, "My clothes don't fit anymore."

While her husband was maintaining an 80-pound weight loss by treating himself as a food addict, his wife had gained about 15 or 20 pounds. Her husband's first thought was, "Ah, I'll have company on this journey, and we can go to support meetings together." His wife, however, had a different idea. She said, "I'm going to have to stop eating between meals, stop eating desserts, and stop having seconds."

Assuming she might be addicted, her husband thought, "Well, that's not likely to happen. I'll give her about a year." He didn't tell her what he was thinking, and that was good because she did give up eating between meals, gave up seconds, and gave up desserts. She lost her weight in a few months, her clothes fit, and for years she had no problem with food. She continued to eat foods that were addictive to her husband and to most food addicts, but she would often say that she didn't have cravings "like my husband used to have."

Those with just simple *obesity* are able to lose weight through diet and exercise with sufficient motivation and support.[130]

EATING DISORDERS

For Emotional Eaters with eating disorders, the problem is lack of coping skills to deal with difficult feelings. For those with binge eating disorder, bulimia, or anorexia, the solution is developing skills to cope with difficult feelings and thoughts without restricting, purging, or bingeing.[131] They are not able to maintain a healthy weight because their major coping mechanism for dealing with difficult feelings is eating comfort foods or engaging in self-abusive food behavior. The solution includes developing effective feeling skills and/or specific therapeutic work to resolve prior emotional trauma.

Harvard faculty conducted a comprehensive U.S. study of the percentage of those currently with eating disorders. This Harvard study is now commonly accepted as the standard for percentages of those with anorexia, bulimia, and binge eating disorder. About 6% of U.S. adult women have a diagnosable eating disorder: .9% are clinically anorexic, 1.5% are chronically bulimic, and 3.5% have binge eating disorder. [132] Many studies show incidences of eating disorders are higher at a sub-clinical level and generally lower for men.

Case Study: Cybil

During adolescence, Cybil, a 5'6" athletic young girl, became preoccupied with her weight. She weighed 115 lbs. and thought she was too fat; her parents disagreed, and there were often fights at home over this issue.

The summer after her junior year, Cybil went away to sports camp and came home having lost about twelve pounds. Her parents were outraged. Cybil argued that there are many different body types and that hers when she was exercising a lot just happened to be particularly thin. She said that she was eating healthily and had built up muscle, which made her appear thinner. This was not convincing to her parents, and they took her to a doctor, who told her that muscle actually weighs more than fat. The argument continued all year. Cybil gained a pound or two and then would lose it again, but she eventually went back up to 115 pounds.

The next year, when her sister was home from college for Christmas, she had a conversation with Cybil and became concerned about how her sister was thinking and talking about her body. On Christmas eve, she suggested that the family do an intervention. Cybil looked still thinner to the family, and she was even more reactive to their feedback about her weight.

At the intervention, all shared their growing concerns. Cybil broke down and cried and said that she thought her family may be right. Her parents said that they would continue paying for her graduate education only if Cybil identified an eating disorder therapist and worked with her until they both thought she didn't need therapeutic support. She agreed.

The outcome was excellent. From this point on, everyone in the family was able to talk about issues of weight and body image and feelings. Cybil continued in therapy for about 16 months, and her weight edged up to the low levels of normal.

Those with *eating disorders* need to deal with the underlying psychological issues, often with therapy, before they are able to consistently control their weight with diet alone. [133]

FOOD SUBSTANCE USE DISORDER

For Food Addicts with a chemical dependency, the problem, as discussed in Denial Statement 3, is physical craving, mental obsession, and addictive personality. Physical craving is like a false starving. Mental obsessions are false thinking believed to be true. Addictive Personality is "self-will run riot" based on distortion of self. The solution is complete abstinence from trigger foods, extraordinary support for obsessive thinking, and transformational or spiritual practice to remedy the distortions of an addictive personality.[134]

Many anorexics are rooted almost exclusively in prior unresolved family trauma, but there is a growing group of anorexics whose restricting is in part or primarily due to a progressive food addiction. We call them anorexic food addicts.

Case Study: Judy

Judy's parents were both drinkers, and her father was a sloppy, unabashed drunk. When he came home with alcohol on his breath, Judy was terrified. At meals, she would put her food on a tray and take it up to her room so as not to be with her father at dinner.

What no one else knew was that Judy was a frequent binger. As she said, "If I opened a package of cookies or a box of doughnuts, it was likely not to be there by the end of the day." She kept the empty wrappers and boxes in a garbage bag in her room.

When she started gaining weight, this terrified her even more than her parents' drinking. She decided that the only way she could control her weight was to stop eating, and that is what she did. (Of course, this was not the only thing she could have done. She could have eaten balanced meals or even just eaten fruits and vegetables. However, this did not occur to her. Since she mostly wanted to eat sugar and flour products, stopping completely seemed perfectly reasonable to her.)

At first, Judy just didn't eat dinner. But soon she was skipping all meals, and her friends, as well as her parents, were mentioning to her how thin she was getting. After about a year, her parents decided she was "dangerously thin," and they began doing everything they could to get her to eat more. Judy's defiance was unexpectedly strong; and within a few months, she had to be hospitalized and force fed.

Out of the hospital, her aunt came to live with her, slowly coaxing her to eat normally, but it didn't last. Finally, after several years of therapy, a new counselor introduced the idea that Judy might be food addicted as well as PTSD, compounded by being an adult child of alcoholics (ACOA).

Many bulimics are also food addicted. While some, like sorority girls in college, take up vomiting to control weight for just a period of time, others, when they decide to stop their bulimic behavior, find that they can't. Like with anorexics, there are some whose difficulty is primarily psychological unresolved trauma, but there is also an important group who are vomiting progressively more times each day to try to contain their progressive food addiction.

The overwhelming majority of food addicts suffer from being overweight or obese. They might have short periods of eating disorder behavior, but the primary reason for their overeating is progressive physical craving, mental obsession, and eventually addictive personality.

Case Study: Joel

Joel had problems sneaking food and lying about it since childhood. He effectively hid his behavior from his parents, but his parents did constantly criticize him for eating too fast and, ironically, praised him for "eating like a man." He always asked for seconds and finished others' food when left on their plates. He was particularly fond of sweet desserts.

Through high school, Joel maintained weight appropriate for his age, mainly because he was so active in sports. He exercised in the morning; and after school, he was usually in organized team play until dinner. Just before graduating from high school, he had his second concussion and was directed by the doctor to cut way back on physical exercise. He began gaining weight.

In college, Joel took up drinking. He never left any alcohol in a glass or a bottle in front of him, but he thought he had as much control as his roommates. What began to be out of control was his eating. At the college cafeteria, Joel selected food on the basis of quantity. There were times when he was eating with a classmate who didn't finish his food, and Joel cleaned the plate for him. At study hall, Joel began to take "energy breaks" every hour. This meant going to the candy dispenser or out to a local fast-food restaurant. By his junior year, Joel was going to the grocery store after dinner to have a supply of binge foods for the evening. He gained over 60 pounds while in college.

When Joel graduated, he needed a physical for a job for which he was applying. The doctor told him his blood pressure and cholesterol were so high that he really was in danger. If he didn't lose weight and keep it off, he was likely to have a heart attack within ten years. The doctor prescribed a pre-diabetic exchange diet or going to Weight Watchers. Joel tried both but couldn't stay with either. Instead of going back to the doctor for more help, he decided the doctor didn't know what he was talking about, and Joel stopped going to the doctor entirely. About ten years later, he had his first heart attack.

In the hospital, Joel told a roommate that he just was not able to stop eating, no matter how hard he tried. His roommate said that he had had the same problem and went to Overeaters Anonymous. It took Joel two years to go to OA, but there he found others with long histories of yo-yo dieting. He heard one person say, "Since grade school, I've either been overeating or on a diet." Joel was also referred to a counselor who understood food addiction.

After a year or so of trial and error, Joel developed a stable food abstinence: no sugar, no flour, no alcohol, and weigh and measure each meal. He also engaged seriously in the spiritual practice of the Twelve Steps and continued to work with a counselor when difficult times or difficult feelings overwhelmed him. He remains at a healthy weight, food abstinent and much happier to this day.

Little current data is available to confirm the extent of food addiction on a national level. Smaller studies have found that the rate in non-clinical samples ranges from an estimated 5 to 26%.[135] Estimates that include clinical samples (i.e., those with diagnosed eating disorders) frequently find higher rates of food addiction.[136] Preliminary food addiction studies provide an educated estimate of the percentages of those overweight and obese people who are food addicted.[137]

The Differences between Dieting and Food Abstinence	
Dieting to Lose Weight	*Abstaining to Be Sober*
1. Assumes you need to take control.	1. Assumes control by will alone is not possible.
2. Works primarily on physical recovery.	2. Works on the mental, emotional, and spiritual recovery as well as the physical.
3. Focuses on putting distractions out of mind.	3. Focuses on sharing thoughts and feelings in the way.
4. The time frame is limited: lose the weight, and you are finished.	4. The time frame is at once one-day-at-a-time for the rest of your life.
5. The best plans are straightforward, science-based and reasonable.	5. The best plans are paradoxical, guided by those who have gone before, and intuitive.
6. The work is a matter of reason and willpower.	6. The work is to gracefully surrender.

© Copyright, Phil Werdell, 1999

Those with a *substance use disorder* or *chemical dependency* on food have an entirely different problem than those who are just eating to "medicate" feelings. Specific addictive food substances actually change the brains of food addicts biochemically such that they start craving and obsessing over the very foods to which they are addicted. Emotional eaters find foods that soothe their feelings, while food addicts find there are foods they "have to eat."[138] Food addicts must completely eliminate these "trigger foods" and, if the disease has progressed, get help to battle their addictive thinking.[139]

We are just beginning to get an educated estimate about how many people are food addicted. Dr. David Kessler, former Director of the U.S. Food and Drug Administration, has estimated that there are 70,000,000 adults in the United States with two unique characteristics of food addiction: physical craving and loss of control.[140] In a National Public Radio interview about his book *The End of Overeating*, Kessler revealed ongoing research in a major metropolitan area indicating that 50% of the obese, 30% of the overweight, and 20% of the "normal" weight adults have these diagnostic features of food addition.[141]

Smaller research projects by doctors about their own practices using the Yale Food Addiction Assessment Scale (YFAS)[142] suggest much more varied numbers: 5%-57% food addicted.[143] How can we reconcile these very large disparities? Of course, one possibility is that there are methodological errors in one or more of the studies. Another possibility: It is still difficult to differentiate a normal eater with weight problems who occasionally binges from someone beginning to develop a serious chemical dependency and substance use disorder. A third possibility is that the YFAS screens just for those who are clinically appropriate for psychiatric treatment, but the larger numbers include those in early stages of food addiction before we would usually authorize treatment for a substance use disorder.

DEMOGRAPHICS

About a third of the U.S. adult population does not have a chronic problem with weight.[144] Those who do generally have three quite different diseases: obesity, eating disorder and chemical dependency on specific food.[145]

A very small percentage of those who are obese are able to lose weight and maintain the weight loss by dieting, but some are able to do this. For example, a study of Weight Watchers found that a substantial percentage were able to lose weight and maintain their weight loss for a year. In a study of all overweight people, including those not using Physicians Weight Loss or commercial diet programs, less than 18% lost weight and maintained it for several years. There is evidence that some of the large percentage were unable to diet successfully because they had eating disorders. There is also evidence that many who could not lose and maintain their weight loss by dieting had a food addiction.

It is obvious, though, that without a clear and correct diagnosis of food addiction, it is not likely that there will be effective treatment.[146] If a doctor prescribes dieting or Weight Watchers to a food addict, the results are likely to be poor. Weight Watchers magazine itself makes this point.[147]

Because most people—even many medical professionals—do not yet fully understand the important difference between these diseases,[148] it is still quite common to make comparisons and to assume moral judgments about those who are supposedly too "weak," "lazy," or "irresponsible."[149] It is important to understand that food addiction is not a moral issue; it is a biochemical disease. Just as cancer once was the focus of irrational shame, food addiction—and other addictions—continue to be so labeled.[150]

Less than 18% of dieters achieve and maintain weight loss for even a year.[151] Twenty percent of those with bariatric surgery do not achieve and maintain weight loss for a year. Moreover, 15-20% of those undergoing bariatric surgery with no prior alcoholism or drug addiction develop clinically significant diagnoses of a substance use disorder with alcohol or drugs within two years.[152]

Although a small percentage of those who are overweight or obese can achieve and maintain weight loss by dieting, most cannot. For some, this is due to eating disorders; for a larger number, this is because of food addiction; and for a majority who are either emotional eaters or food addicts, they have both. They have lost control of their eating to various degrees; but none should be compared with normal eaters, who are able to lose weight through diet and exercise. None should be shamed or blamed; they should be referred to food addiction professionals or to support groups which are effective in helping food addicts.

Most food addiction is still misdiagnosed and mistreated; this creates further problems.[153] Food addicts hear doctors say that they must diet or that they must engage in a certain line of therapy. Food addicts work as hard as possible following directions. If they are unsuccessful, they often take on guilt and shame, especially if the health professional says or implies that they have not followed medical advice. This is another case of blaming the victim, and if it is done over a period of years—which it often is—it can create a serious problem of internalized oppression for the overweight food addict. This internalized shame can become as serious a problem as overweight and other secondary medical effects of food addiction.

FOOD ADDICTION DENIAL
NO.6

<u>Denial Statement #6</u>: "If someone has lost control over their eating, they should go to a therapist or eating disorder specialist to resolve 'underlying issues.'"

<u>Rebuttal</u>: For those who have an eating disorder – and <u>only</u> an eating disorder – this is true; they do lose their excess weight and/or shed abusive eating behaviors after therapy and often return to being normal eaters. However, many who have a clinical diagnosable eating disorder <u>also</u> have a substance use disorder regarding specific food(s), i.e., food addiction.[154] These people also need an abstinence-based treatment using the addictive model. Moreover, there are still more whose correct diagnosis is food addiction rather than an eating disorder. For those with food addiction, therapy focused on underlying issues can actually be counterproductive in that it increases denial regarding food-related substance use disorder.

CHAPTER 6

EATING DISORDERS VS. FOOD ADDICTION

The appropriate treatment for the 10% of Americans[155] who have a clinical-level eating disorder is development of emotional skills and resolution of prior trauma towards a goal of being able to eat all foods in moderation.[156] However, the 2013 Fifth Edition of the American Psychiatric Association (APA) Diagnostic and Statistical Manual of Mental Disorders (DSM-5) finds that:

> "Some individuals with [eating] disorders report eating-related symptoms resembling those typically endorsed by individuals with substance use disorders such as physical craving and patterns of compulsive use."[157]

In short, some of those with Anorexia, Bulimia, or Binge Eating Disorder are also appropriately diagnosed with food addiction.

If a person is both eating disordered and food addicted, using the psychological treatment for food addiction alone will not work.

- **Food addicts should not be encouraged to eat all foods in moderation.** Treatment begins by identifying foods that trigger binges and eliminating them completely. This may mean having to go through a period of withdrawal during detoxification.[158]

- **The food addict is not able to do intuitive eating.** A food addict should not be expected to learn the difference between emotional hunger and physical hunger until binge foods are removed. Rather, the food addict must be taught that physical cravings are different from natural physical hunger; and cravings created by the disease overpower or anesthetize the food addict to normal and healthy feelings. Also, with middle- and late-stage food addicts, cognitive behavioral therapy is usually insufficient.[159]

- **Progressive biochemical denial in food addiction must be challenged.** A diagnosis from a health professional is insufficient. Food addicts themselves must understand and accept that they are chemically dependent; and if they are at a critical stage, they need extraordinary support over the long term.[160]

- **Food addiction is a chronic disease.** Cravings return if addictive foods are reintroduced. Mental obsessions about foods are not exclusively from lack of cognitive and emotional skill or prior trauma; they are from biochemical changes in the brain.[161]

The following chart shows the difference between eating disorder therapy and food addiction recovery work.

DIFFERENCE BETWEEN EATING DISORDER THERAPY AND FOOD ADDICTION RECOVERY WORK	
Traditional Eating Disorder Therapy	*Food Addiction Recovery Work*
Traditional eating disorder therapy assumes the problem is not the food.	Food addiction recovery work assumes the problem is the food, until it is not the food. Then, it is not the food.
It works primarily on mental-emotional healing.	It begins with physical abstinence and then mental, emotional, and spiritual healing.
It is usually led by someone who is academically trained in eating disorder therapy and professionally licensed.	A majority of the work is done in peer-support groups with groups led by recovering food addicts. When needed, there are also groups led by food addiction professionals.
The time frame is limited: When you develop skills to deal with irrational thoughts and unresolved feelings, you are finished.	The timeframe is paradoxical: The focus is on being abstinent and in recovery one day at a time, and recovery often continues for one's entire life.
The counselor or therapist is seen as the primary authority.	The ultimate authority is seen as God, *as each person sees God,* often as expressed in the group conscience.

When a person is both clinically eating disordered and a critical-stage food addict, treatment is complicated. Both diseases must be treated, sometimes alternating between one and the other. For late-stage food addicts, the rule is to begin with the addiction model and treat difficult emotions as they come up.

We will now examine each of the major eating disorders and how they are sometimes connected to food addiction.

Binge Eating and Food Addiction: How are they connected?

In the past, there was considerable controversy about whether those who overate were doing it for psychological reasons or were eating out of a chemical dependency. We now know that both can be true, and for many overeaters—probably a large majority—both social-environmental and biochemical addictive factors are in play.

We find it useful to call a trauma-based problem an eating disorder and a chemical dependency problem a food addiction. Some have just one—binge eating disorder (BED) or substance use disorder with food (SUD). Those whose diseases are most advanced are usually referred to as "double winners," meaning they suffer from both diseases. If both diseases are not treated, these "double winners" chronically relapse.

Those with primarily binge eating disorder tend to talk about themselves as "emotional eaters." They "go to their comfort foods" in times of stress. One way of looking at their eating disorder is that they have come to rely on specific foods, or food in general, as their major coping mechanism to deal with difficult feelings. Unlike healthy eaters with good feeling skills, binge eaters will often know the major types of situations which will trigger eating and the specific food drugs that are their "comfort foods." Treatment is to develop other coping skills for dealing with difficult feelings.

Those with primarily food addiction tend to talk about eating as one of their favorite activities in life. They "live to eat," and they often binge when they are feeling happy or excited as well as when they are feeling sad, angry or afraid. One way of looking at a food addiction is as a condition of "false starving." Unlike normal eaters, food addicts don't just feel hungry, they also have a feeling that life would not be worth living without certain foods and/or they have a sense that they will die if they don't eat more right now! They overeat even when they have clearly had enough food to satisfy their nutritional needs. In later stages, they overeat even when their over-eating has made them feel very uncomfortable. The treatment is eliminat-ing the toxic foods completely and then working through the underlying emotional and spiritual problems caused by the disease.

Since most of those with advanced binge eating disorder are also food addicted, however, the language used to describe the experience is not always useful in clarifying what the problem really is. In fact, many profes-sionals use the words "binge eating," "compulsive overeating," and "food addiction" interchangeably, and this does not provide enough information for an accurate diagnosis.

Why is this distinction important? Because the essential treatment for each can be very different.

Those with a binge eating disorder alone focus on feelings and on issues of cognitive behavioral therapy. The fundamental idea is that "it is not what you eat, but what is eating you." The goal is to work through rigid, irrational thinking; focus on developing better eating behaviors or habits; and practice dealing with feelings directly without using food. Regarding food, the goal is to learn to be able to eat a balanced, nutritious diet and be able to eat all foods in moderation.

In contrast, those who are food addicted need to begin by eliminat-ing toxic foods completely, then doing the underlying mental-emotional and spiritual work necessary to maintain this food abstinence over the long term. The initial goal is to detoxify from the food(s) to which the food addict is chemically dependent. More advanced food addicts then need to deal with their addictive minds: euphoric recall, compulsive thinking about food, and mental obsessions related to eating. Beginning with the breaking down of denial, the long-term goal is a personality change, or spiritual experience, and ability to accept help from others and a Higher Power to deal with a food addict's powerlessness over food.

Of course, as we have said, the more common situation is for binge eaters to develop an addiction and for those who are food addicted from birth to also have plenty of childhood trauma. In these cases, you treat the part of the problem that is most advanced. When someone is equally addicted and emotionally disabled, the rule of thumb is always to start with the food addiction, then work on emotional healing whenever it is necessary to maintain physical abstinence and recovery.

The difficult question is usually this: When a person has a diagnosable binge eating disorder, is the person also food addicted?

At this time, the most frequent way people find out whether or not they are food addicted is by finding out that over a period of time, treatments as a normal eater (i.e., dieting) or emotional eater (i.e., eating disorder therapy) have not worked. A common pattern is: Diets do not work, so they go to a counselor. After a year or more, therapy does not work, so they go to a food Twelve Step fellowship. If this works, that is good.

But what if someone is not able to achieve and maintain physical food abstinence using the Twelve Steps? If this were an alcoholic or drug addict in AA, the person would be referred to a one-week detox. If that was not enough, then it would be followed by a 28-day treatment program and possibly further time in a halfway house. The problem is that in the entire country, there are only a very small number of such programs for food addiction.[162] There are no hospital-based primary treatment centers at all since insurance funding was cut off in the late 1990s.

Assessment instruments are now available to diagnose possible food addiction at earlier stages. The Twelve Step programs all have self-assessment questions.[163] There is an assessment schedule for normal eaters, emotional eaters, and food addicts in *Bariatric Surgery and Food Addiction:*

Preoperative Considerations.[164] The only peer-reviewed assessment instrument is the YALE Food Addiction Assessment Scale.[165] The most in-depth assessment procedure is using the UNCOPE[166] screening tool followed by the interview-based SUGAR[167] assessment.

Bulimia and Food Addiction: How are they connected?

How do we know if someone is bulimic? The answer is fairly straightforward.

- Do they binge and purge?

- Do they keep doing this after they have decided to stop?

- Do they physically vomit food, even when they are not sick?

- Do they use pills, ipecac, laxatives, or diuretics to control their weight?

- Do they exercise excessively, sometimes even to the point of hurting themselves?

- Do they do highly restrictive dieting over and over again?

These are the common physical characteristics of bulimia.[168]

For our purposes, there are basically two types of bulimics. The first type of bulimic has a high degree of body distortion, often thinks they are fat when they are not. They are extremely afraid of being fat and purge ritualistically when they think they have ingested too many calories. There is often a psychological component, and the purging can be a coping mechanism for releasing difficult feelings.

The second type of bulimic is food addicted and is purging to try to control the results of out-of-control eating. One simple indication of food-addicted bulimia is that they had a history of bingeing on foods before they started purging. The second common characteristic is that the person cycles between out-of-control eating and out-of-control purging and getting fat. The most important characteristic for food-addicted bulimics is that most of their bingeing is on commonly addictive foods, e.g., added sugar, flour, excess fat, etc. When these foods are eliminated, the bingeing also stops, there is no more reason to purge, and they do not purge. Of course, some bulimics are of both types; they binge and purge due to prior psychological problems and because they have become chemically dependent on specific foods. They need to be treated for both diseases.

Anorexia and Food Addiction—
How are they connected?

The common misconception regarding food addicts is that they are all overweight. Many bulimics look like they are at healthy weight even though they have very unhealthy thoughts and feelings, but it is important to notice that even some people who are underweight are food addicted.

Anorexia is traditionally understood as a psycho-social disorder.[169] For our purposes here, however, there are three types of anorexia.

The first type of anorexia is often viewed as a compensating measure to deal with highly conflicted family situations in early childhood. The child has trouble asserting any control in the family, so he or she begins to focus on controlling their weight. When family members become concerned that the child is too thin, it is almost impossible to make them eat. The child experiences success; moreover, in many industrially developed countries, there are distorted sexist values for hyper-thin women and some men. So children now see themselves as successful not only in the family, but in terms of larger social norms.

The second type of anorexia develops in response to food addiction. It is sometimes called anorexic food addiction. Like the food-addicted bulimic, anorexics of this type usually have a history of eating out of control and gaining weight before their practice of over-restricting becomes dangerous. This double diagnosis of anorexia and food addiction is important because treatment must include complete abstinence from major binge foods as well as psychological treatment regarding disordered thinking and stress from prior unresolved trauma. It is especially common to miss the diagnosis of food addiction in anorexic food addicts. However, if the food addiction is not diagnosed and treated, these people will continually relapse. They will have physical cravings and mental obsessions leading them to feel they have to overeat. If they do begin to overeat and get fat, this, of course, will retrigger the anorexia.

The third type of anorexia is one in which a person becomes addicted to the feeling of being in control. It is actually the illusion of control. A person who is preoccupied with food and weight and has a highly rigid form of restricting which leads to malnourishment is not really in control. This form of anorexia is treated as an addictive disease as exemplified by the fellowship Anorexics and Bulimics Anonymous (ABA).[170] In this model of anorexia, an adrenalin-like internal drug becomes addictive; ABA calls the drug of choice the "illusion of control."[171]

How can an anorexic be food addicted? Quite simply, they alternate between overeating and over-restricting. One obvious sign is a history of out-of-control eating—usually bingeing, sometimes purging, and almost always becoming overweight by traditional medical standards. For these anorexic food addicts, restricting foods in the extreme, sometimes not eating at all for days, is a way of compensating for a binge. Then regular fasting becomes a strategy for periodic weight loss after gaining by overeating. It is only as the anorexia progresses that such a person stays thin—and then becomes unhealthily thin—and begins to "look like an anorexic."

A second indication that an anorexic is chemically dependent on food is if the person fantasizes excessively about normally addictive foods, especially sweets and "junk foods." As with bulimics, if there is a history of craving sugar, flour, and fat, this is a reason to consider the possibility of food addiction as a second diagnosis.

All anorexics obsess about their bodies and fear getting fat. It is less known that many anorexics also obsess about food. This often manifests as precise and compulsive calorie counting, a list—often quite long—of "bad foods," and a preoccupation with eating in a way that they can control what they do—and more importantly, *do not* put in their mouths. What is less common is a constant or frequent idea about wanting to eat sweets, snack foods, or just "more" of any food. Especially if this latter obsession gets so strong that it seems like "I just have to have" that food, there is good reason to assume this person is food addicted as well as anorexic.

In general, it is our experience that people with advanced anorexia and food addiction need more time and support to recover than those who are only chemically dependent on food. Anorexia has its own denial, **and** the food-addicted anorexic can have special problems breaking food-addictive denial. The illusion of control in anorexia—and often bulimia—makes people who were anorexic and bulimic in their youth become compulsive overeaters in adulthood. If they are food addicted, they often need a great deal of help to break through their biochemical food-dependent denial.[172]

* * * * *

In conclusion, all of those who suffer from the various eating disorders of anorexia, bulimia, and binge eating disorder cannot be successfully treated just by working on underlying psychological issues. If they are also food addicted, this co-diagnosis must also be treated; and the treatment of both diseases at once can be essential to long-term recovery.

FOOD ADDICTION DENIAL
NO. 7

Denial Statement #7: "There is no evidence that food addiction can be treated effectively."

Rebuttal: The basic principles of treatment for addiction are complete elimination of all chemically dependent substances, extraordinary support for addiction as a brain disease, and some form of long-term transformational spiritual practice.[173] These are the principles for the treatment of food addiction.[174]

A growing body of research indicates that early-, middle-, and late-stage food addicts can be effectively treated using the addiction model. Outcome research includes: 1) thousands of anecdotal stories for early-stage food addicts diminishing or ending craving and overeating by eliminating trigger foods; 2) seven self-studies of food-related Twelve Step organizations, many members of which were mostly middle- and late-stage food addicts; and 3) three outcome research studies for professional treatment of late- and final-stage food addicts—a residential hospital-based program, a residential workshop-based program, and an outpatient program.[175]

CHAPTER 7

EFFECTIVE TREATMENT
THE ADDICTION TREATMENT MODEL

Food addiction is a physical, mental-emotional and spiritual problem. This requires a physical, mental-emotional and spiritual solution. The basic principles of effective treatment are:

1. Eliminate foods that trigger physical cravings and out-of-control eating behaviors,

2. Develop support to accept food addiction as a brain disease and to cope with mental obsessions,

3. Practice a discipline which removes blocks to self-esteem and enhances spiritual progress.[176]

There are many ways of doing this, and the intensity of the treatment depends on the progression of the disease.[177]

Food Addiction—Progression and Recommended Actions

Disease Stage	Recommended Actions
Pre-Disease	**Prevention**
No sign of abnormal eating or reactions to specific foods. If no dependency or pathology develops, this stage will continue through the person's entire life.	Education about food addiction. Ongoing checks for signs of chemical dependency. Moderation in eating, especially commonly addictive foods, e.g., sugar, caffeine, excess fat, alcohol, drugs.
Early Stage	**Detox and Abstinence**
Problems with weight management, cycles of weight gain followed by dieting, weight loss, and weight gain again. Occasional binge eating on sugar, excess fat, or volume. Could be early-stage food addiction or a normal eater making unhealthy choices.	Identify addictive foods. Eliminate binge and trigger foods. Move through detoxification. This often seems extreme if negative consequences are not yet severe, an early stage of addictive denial.
Middle Stage	**Twelve-Step Group/Counselor**
Frequent binge eating and grazing. Purging or severe restriction may begin. Rationalizing before eating, guilt afterward. Could be advancing food addiction or emotional problem eater with a psychologically based eating disorder.	Participation in a food-related Twelve-Step program, e.g., Overeaters Anonymous, and/or work with a food addictions counselor. Assistance with addressing blocks to physical abstinence, especially denial. Develop feeling skills, resolve trauma.
Late Stage	**More Structure and Support**
Serious consequences from overeating—morbid obesity, Type II diabetes, chronic depression and/or spiritual disillusionment, and eating anyway. Food no longer provides comfort, escape, oblivion, etc. Loss of control, increasing tolerance.	Participation in a highly structured Twelve-Step program, e.g., Food Addicts in Recovery Anonymous, Compulsive Eaters Anonymous—HOW. Outpatient treatment and/or workshops such as those offered by ACORN (now SHiFT, Recovery by Acorn). Abstinence as a spiritual path.
Final Stage	**Primary Inpatient or Residential Treatment**
Severe consequences—hospitalization for heart attacks, suicide attempts, lost jobs or inability to work, ruined relationships, treatment and/or intestinal surgery followed by relapse, housebound or confined to nursing homes.	Given the lack of any hospital-based inpatient treatment for food addiction, alternatives include Turning Point of Tampa, Milestones, Shades of Hope, ACORN's multi-year program. This is sometimes insufficient.
DEATH	

© copyright Phil Werdell, *Bariatric Surgery & Food Addiction: Preoperative Considerations*, 2008 [178]

Early-Stage Recovery

In *early-stage* food addiction, treatment tends to be mainly physical: eliminating binge foods and self-abusive food behaviors. The problem is that complete abstinence from favored foods often seems too extreme compared to people's perceived understanding of the addiction. Social support makes a major difference. For example, the Church of the Seventh Day Adventists prescribes avoidance of added sugar, and most members are compliant with the active support of family and parishioners.[179] The Browns Mill Elementary School in Lithonia, Georgia, eliminated all sugar in vending machines and in the lunchroom and asked parents to support sugar-free eating at home; the students, teachers, and families got behind this principle, and there were positive results.[180] Therapeutic food addiction recovery groups[181] and peer mutual support groups like food-related Twelve Step fellowships[182] often create enough support for people to achieve and maintain abstinence.

Anecdotal Case Studies: Individual stories about people with the symptom of food addiction and success in treating the problem using an addiction model are often considered minimally relevant scientifically; but now the number of such case studies has grown to a statistically significant point in terms of showing that some people who are overweight can be effectively treated as food addicts.

It is not unusual now to meet people casually who call themselves food addicts, have stopped eating all sugary items, and have been generally successful regarding their weight.

The Uber Driver

Because of my eyesight, I have not been able to drive for over ten years, and I frequently use Uber. In about half of these situations, I will strike up some small talk, and the driver will ask, "What do you do for a living?" When I tell them I work with food addicts, about half the time, they say, "I should be dealing with that problem." Frequently the person is overweight and has had trouble dieting, especially maintaining weight loss after losing. This is an indication for me that there are many more possible early-stage food addicts than we normally believe. But sometimes the driver will explain that what works for them is to stop eating sweets altogether or to avoid fast foods or junk foods. Here, the solution is specifically not moderation, but abstinence, and is an indication that that person might not only be food addicted, but might also have found an effective way of treating the disease in their own.

Nurse Lucy

I recently went for day surgery, and the pre-op nurse asked me if I had any allergies. I told her I was addicted to sugar and did not want glucose drip during the operation or any foods with sugar or flour upon coming out of anesthesia. She said, "Oh, I fast from chocolate." What she meant was that over a couple of years she found that she could never eat just one piece of chocolate, and that sometimes she would actually have the thought of eating the whole box. While she never had an extreme binge, her lack of control really bothered her. As a very health-conscious nurse, knowing that added sugar at that level was not that good for her anyway, she tried to moderate her chocolate use. When she couldn't do this, she decided to just stop eating chocolate entirely. This worked so well that she hadn't had chocolate for several years. Nurse Lucy had never heard of the concept of food addiction and didn't use the words "food abstinence," but she definitely had the characteristics of early-stage food addiction, and she certainly was abstaining from her specific binge food.

As of this writing, the Twelve Step group Overeaters Anonymous (OA) has published two volumes of short recovery stories from their membership to which researchers have easy access, a total of more than fifty case studies of compulsive overeaters.[183] The OA members tend to be middle- and late-stage food addicts; but beyond this, the collections are proof that food addiction is a very "democratic" disease. Stories are of young people and older people; a majority of white women, but also men, Afro-Americans and Hispanics; those who got really heavy, and those who are "normal" weight by abuse purging or exercise or diet pills; those who are gay, and those who are straight; those who purge, and those who don't; those who have also been anorexic, and so forth. The problem with the OA stories is that there is no clear distinction between those who are food addicted and those who just have a trauma-based eating disorder. About two-thirds have several characteristics of food addiction, and a majority present as having both a clinical eating disorder and a substance use disorder regarding specific foods.

A newer fellowship, Food Addicts in Recovery Anonymous (FA), published a similar volume with thirty such stories—"What I was like in the disease? what happened? and what it is like now?" This is particularly useful to researchers in that it separates the self-identified food addicts from other overeaters, and almost all members have the same definition of food abstinence and use a very similar food plan.[184] They commit their food specifically each day to a peer sponsor; and they accept as requirements the suggestion to attend at least two meetings, do reading and writing on the program's literature, and help other food addicts with less recovery experience. This profile is similar to those of special movements within OA focusing on the addiction model and to other newer, smaller independent food-related fellowships.[185] There are over 100 more "recovery stories" in past issues of the monthly FA magazine, *the connection*.

Also available are many more detailed food addiction recovery stories, as well as a growing number of book-length memoirs of self-described food addicts. Some examples:

- The story of a "typical" middle-aged overeater is chronicled in Nancy Appleton's *Suicide by Sugar.*[186]

- Eve Schaub authored her own memoir about her *Year of No Sugar.*[187]

- For a memoir from a man's point of view, in his *Fat Boy, Thin Man,*[188] Michael Prager tells of his journey to food addiction recovery and to losing 160 pounds and keeping it off for over twenty years.

- M. Bullitt-Jonas, living with her administrator father on the Harvard University campus, tells of her recovery in *Holy Hunger: A Woman's Journey from Food Addiction to Spiritual Fulfillment.*[189]

- Compulsive overeating recovery stories of Native American women and men can be found in *The Red Road to Wellbriety in the Native American Way.*[190]

- Burt Nordstrand, a successful businessman who was also multi-addicted, writes of his coming to peace with alcoholism and drug addiction as well as food addiction in *Living with the Enemy: An Explorations of Addiction and Recovery.*[191]

- Debbie Danowski, who had to go to in-patient treatment for food addiction, describes her experience in *Locked Up for Eating Too Much.*[192]

- A compulsive eater contrasted with the stories of those other addicted in *America Anonymous,* by Benoit Denizet-Lewis.[193]

- Dr. Joan Ifland recorded the stories of a group of overeating obese adults and found that each of them had many of the major characteristics of substance use disorder and also sometimes characteristics of alcoholism and drug addiction.[194]

- A Christian who integrated her Biblical teachings with Twelve Step practices in *Sweet Surrender: Christian 12 Step Recovery from Food Addiction.*[195]

- Raja Batareseh's *My Yellow Suit: A Lifelong Quest to lose Weight and Gain Happiness,*[196] the first publicly identified Middle Easterner food addict. (The English version only described her powerlessness over dieting; the following Arabic edition adds her food addition recovery solution.)

Stories in OA and FA publications.

- **No Contradicting Evidence:** The Brownell and Gold graduate textbook *Food and Addiction: A Comprehensive Handbook* provides updated corroborating research. Also, in his 2017 bestseller *The Case Against Sugar,* Gary Taubes begins by presenting dozens of current studies regarding sugar and evidence of food addiction. The most recent confirmation is by Dr. Mark Hyman, *Food: What the Heck Should I Eat?*[197]

Clinical Impressions.

If the self-report and judgments of food addicts themselves are suspect, then we add a level of objectivity and expertise by finding out what physicians, dieticians, therapists, and other clinicians observe.

A number of therapists and physicians have written books about ways they have helped their patients deal with food addiction. Each of these books includes short or long case studies of people diagnosed with and successfully treated for food addiction.[198]

Studies of Outcomes for Food Related Twelve Step Programs

Historical Context

Obesity rates have doubled worldwide since 1980, according to research published in the journal *The Lancet* (Feb 4, 2011). In 1980, 4.8% of men and 7.9% of women were obese. Those percentages jumped to 9.8% of men and 13.8% of women in 2008.[199] It was a serious medical problem, but not yet the epidemic it is today. There were many popular diets, and some of those who kept regaining the weight went to counseling to work on underlying psychological issues. In this case, quite a few were not helped with their weight problem in the long term.

In 1960, one such middle-age woman in Los Angeles was watching the late-night talk shows—and eating. She saw a hooded man from Gamblers Anonymous being interviewed. This man had found a solution to his out-of-control betting problem. As she heard the progression of his gambling disease, she realized that she overate the same way he had gambled. With his help, she and a neighbor friend started a Twelve Step program for overeaters in the model of Alcoholics Anonymous (AA). They called it Overeaters Anonymous.

About the same time in Texas, a longtime recovered alcoholic was suffering badly from his chronic obesity. He wondered if the AA program that had helped him put down the booze completely might help him with his loss of control over food. He started Gluttons Anonymous. Soon there were five Gluttons recovery groups in Texas, and they joined with the eight overeating groups in California for a first world conference. With each group getting one vote, they elected (8 to 5) that all groups be named Overeaters Anonymous (OA).[200]

From the beginning, there were two informal factions in OA. One group with long experiences in therapy thought of their problem as primarily one of underlying psychological issues; they thought that food abstinence meant not eating between planned moderate meals. The other group came mostly from AA; they saw their problem as an addiction and began by asking what specific food(s) they needed to eliminate completely. The first food plan, mimeographed on grey paper, was called the Grey Sheet, and it eliminated all sugar or grain. There was also an Orange Sheet and many other varieties of written diets. Others preferred working toward the ability to intuitively choose healthy foods. Soon, anorexics, bulimics, and binge eaters were encouraged to join. From the beginning, OA was very diverse, everyone deciding for themselves what food plan to use, some using no food plan at all.[201] What united all members and groups was the spiritual program of the Twelve Steps.[202]

The program worked almost immediately for some members, but others struggled for years. Among those seeing themselves as food addicts, specialized meetings began throughout the country which experimented with more structure. The "suggestions" in the general program were tried as "requirements." Some meetings focused on everyone's using the Grey Sheet food plan. Members began each sharing with a statement about being committed to putting their food abstinence first: "No matter what."

A movement within OA called OA-HOW required a surrendered food plan with no sugar, flour, or alcohol, with each meal committed to a sponsor and weighed and measured. HOW required three phone calls and a writing assignment each day, participation in at least two meetings a week, and readings from the AA literature for the first 80 days.

Another movement within OA suggested members just listen during meetings until they have 90 days of abstinence. The idea was that meetings should be about how people had recovered, and problems could be discussed outside or with a sponsor. These were called OA 90-Day Meetings.

There were also special meetings for bulimics, for those needing a 100-pound weight loss, for women, and for studying the Twelve Steps. There were speakers' meetings, topic meetings, writing meetings, meditation meetings. The distinction between emotional eaters and food addicts—or both—ran through all these different meetings. The diversity in the fellowship seemed to really be working. By 1980, there were 3,906 meetings worldwide and an estimated 55,000 active members in OA.[203]

- In the 1990s, those OA members and groups with a strict definition of their disease started to break off and form entirely separate fellowships.

- A group seeing themselves as food addicted using Kay Sheppard's writing and food plan broke off in Florida and formed Food Addicts Anonymous (FAA).

- Some of the members in OA-HOW decided they just wanted the support of food addicts and formed Compulsive Eaters Anonymous-HOW (CEA-HOW) on the West Coast.

- For similar reasons, the founders of OA 90-Day Meetings formed the separate fellowship Food Addicts in Recovery Anonymous (FA).

- OA Grey Sheet format dominated most of the OA meetings in New York, and they led the formation of GreySheeters Anonymous (GreySheet).

As of this writing, the membership of OA is over 50,000. However, the active membership of all food-related Twelve Step organizations totals over 75,000 members.

Although not discussed in this writing, members and groups with emotional eating tendencies also founded separate fellowships.[204] One new organization used the general content of the Twelve Steps, but recast them in the Christian context.[205] There were/are also several organizations which were/are used by food addicts for their own healing but did/do not use the Twelve Steps at all.[206] All of these separate organizations have become worldwide fellowships. We focus on the food addiction emphasis.

Outcome Studies

Overeaters Anonymous (OA) conducted research on random/selective samples of their membership in 1981, 1992, 2002, 2010, and 2017. Food Addicts in Recovery Anonymous (FA) conducted similar rigorous research in 2011 and 2016. There was also a study of OA by independent outside researcher Kerri-Lynn Murphy Kriz in 2002. The sampling methods differ from study to study, but they are generally comparable.

Demographics: The sample groups in all eight studies have many similar characteristics. About 90% are female and 10% male. Though from many countries, over 95% are English speaking. A large majority self-describe as white, with FA having a slightly larger percentage people of color. They tend to be middle aged and older, though there are some young people. About half have college degrees – AA, BA, MA, and PHD, more with college experience. Demographics across studies are quite consistent.

Recovery Outcomes: With food addiction, weight loss and maintaining a healthy weight are secondary outcomes to eliminating physical craving and mental obsession. However, health professionals and the general public tend to view weight loss as the most important outcome, so we include this information, along with the data about food addiction abstinence.

In the five self-studies of Overeaters Anonymous, the questions listing weight loss data are slightly different from survey to survey.

- In <u>OA Survey I (1981)</u>, the average non-new member reported an *average weight loss since entering of 31.4 pounds* with an average abstinence from compulsive eating of 2.6 months; *24.4% reported reaching a healthy weight and maintaining that for an average of 2.2 years*; 87.7% reported smaller weight loss fluctuations prior to OA.[207]

- In <u>OA Survey 2 (1992)</u> on the key issue of weight, there were self-reports of "substantial average weight loss." Respondents reported *an average 40.8-pound weight loss since joining OA and an average of 3.97 years for which the loss was maintained.*[208]

- In <u>OA Study 3 (2002)</u>, most of those who responded said that they experienced improvements in eating behavior: little or none (5.0%), moderate (15.4%), significant (45.6%), and maintaining abstinence, (33.7%); *46% said they had achieved a healthy body weight* since joining; and, significantly for those food addicted, *56% found their food obsession lifted.*[209]

- In <u>OA Survey 4 (2010)</u>, the *average weight loss was 45 pounds, with 51% currently maintaining a healthy weight*; 78% had relapsed at some point; 82% continued attending meetings during relapse.[210]

- In <u>OA Survey 5 (2017)</u>, again, the *average weight loss was 45 pounds,* but *54% were maintaining healthy weight; 73% reported having lost weight*; 82% had relapsed at some point; 84% continued attending meetings during relapse.[211]

Thus, according to the published OA self-studies, <u>there seems to have been an increase over the decades in the amount of average weight loss and in the length of time weight loss was maintained</u>, though slight, over the last two studies. If the OA samples represent the outcomes in the organization as a whole, the results of working this food-related Twelve Step program are better than for most diets, even though previously, most of the members of OA have been unsuccessful at many diets and weight loss programs.[212]

This is confirmed by an outside study by Kriz, which found that <u>some adults previously eating out of control and then working the OA program can have a substantial weight loss and maintain it on average more than the outcomes of most diet programs</u>.[213]

In the two self-studies by Food Addicts in Recovery Anonymous, the data is comparable.

- In the FA 2011 study, 93% lost weight since joining FA.[214]
- In the FA 2016 study, 96% reported weight loss and had reported being at goal weight for five or more years.[215]

The charts of the 2016 study contain a more detailed breakdown.

Q13: From the time you joined FA to the present, please indicate your weight loss or gain in FA:	
178	None 4.31%
36	Had to gain weight 0.87%
761	Lost 1-25 lbs. 18.43%
1080	Lost 26-50 lbs. 26.16%
858	Lost 51-75 lbs. 20.78%
567	Lost 76-100 lbs. 13.73%
286	Lost 101-125 lbs. 6.93%
141	Lost 126-150 lbs. 3.41%
93	Lost 151-200 lbs. 2.25%
30	Lost over 200 lbs. 0.73%
99	No Answer 2.40%
4129	Total 100.00%

Q10: Please indicate how long you have followed the disciplines of FA:	
0	Not currently abstinent .... .00%
819	Less than 90 days 19.84%
789	90 days-1 year 19.11%
840	13 months-2 years 20.34%
794	3-5 years 19.23%
575	6-10 years 13.93%
150	11-15 years 3.63%
26	16-20 years 0.63%
26	21-30 years 0.63%
6	More than 30 years 0.15%
104	No Answer 2.52%
4129	Total 100.00%

Q11: Please indicate how long you have had back-to-back abstinence (as defined by FA):	
313	Not currently abstinent 7.58%
1260	Less than 90 days 30.52%
965	90 days-1 year 23.37%
653	13 months-2 years 15.81%
494	3- 5 years 11.96%
243	6-10 years 5.89%
76	11-15 years 1.84%
14	16-20 years 0.34%
11	21-30 years 0.27%
2	More than 30 years 0.05%
98	No Answer 2.37%
4129	Total 100.00%

The weight loss outcomes and the results of abstinence regarding specific addictive foods are better in FA than in OA for three possible reasons. First, OA does not make a distinction in its survey data between those who are food addicts and those who are not. Second, there is a common understanding in OA that the weight loss and abstinence outcomes are much higher in the movements within the organization—OA Greysheet, OA-HOW, and OA 90-Day Meetings—than in the rest of the fellowship, which is less structured and does not rigorously define itself as addictive. Third, long-time members of OA 90-Day were founders of FA, and this may substantially increase the numbers of those with long-term abstinence in FA.

Probably most important in terms of the effectiveness of Twelve Step treatment are the health benefits for working an OA or FA program.

In some of the OA surveys, there is also information about other health questions. For example:

In the 0A 1992 Survey, top ways OA members saw their lives improved by OA:

- Emotional health   93%
- Spiritual life   92%
- Less food preoccupation 81%
- Family life   79%
- Physical health   72%

Of those reporting with the following medical problems, the percentage of reporting progress since OA included:

- Emotional problems   93%
- Diabetes   87%
- High blood pressure   86%
- Hypoglycemia   85%
- Stomach problems   81%

In the 2002 OA Survey, for those food addicted, 56% found their food obsession lifted.

The 2010 OA Survey contained a life-improvements chart:

Life Improvements					
	Significant Improvement	Moderate Improvement	A little Improvement	No Improvement	Was not an Issue
Daily functioning	63%	20%	9%	3%	5%
Overall physical health	50%	28%	12%	6%	4%
Mental/emotional health	72%	19%	6%	2%	1%
Spiritual connection	70%	17%	7%	3%	3%
Weight issues	49%	25%	14%	9%	3%
Relationships	56%	25%	10%	4%	5%

In the 2017 OA Survey, between 80%-90% of OAs claimed improvement in mental/emotional health (94%), daily functioning (93%), spiritual connection (92%), relationships (88%), and overall physical health (84%), as well as weight issues (80%). The following life improvement chart was also included in the 2017 survey:

Life Improvements			
	Significant Improvement	Moderate Improvement	Total
Mental/emotional health	76%	18%	94%
Daily functioning	72%	21%	93%
Spiritual connection	74%	18%	92%
Relationships	64%	24%	88%
Overall physical health	58%	26%	84%
Weight issues	53%	27%	80%

The 2011 FA survey included detailed answers to questions most asked by physicians, dieticians, psychiatrists, therapists, and other allied health professionals. In particular, the question was asked, "Have you, with the help of your health care professionals, been able to discontinue any medications since FA? Answering yes were 29%; 58% answered no; and 13% had no answer. Other information in the FA survey included:

Q13: From the time you joined FA to the present, please indicate your weight loss or gain in FA:

178	None	4.31%
36	Had to gain weight	0.87%
761	Lost 1-25 lbs	18.43%
1080	Lost 26-50 lbs	26.16%
858	Lost 51-75 lbs	20.78%
567	Lost 76-100 lbs	13.73%
286	Lost 101-125 lbs	6.93%
141	Lost 126-150 lbs	3.41%
93	Lost 151-200 lbs	2.25%
30	Lost over 200 lbs	0.73%
99	No Answer	2.40%
4129	Total	100.00%

Q14: Has FA abstinence helped with any health issues? Please mark all that apply.

3368	Yes	81.57%
761	No	18.43%
4129	Total	100.00%
1334	Anxiety	32.31%
257	Asthma	6.22%
114	Bi-Polar Disorder	2.76%
1484	Depression	35.94%
559	Diabetes	13.54%
778	Gastrointestinal disorders	18.84%
1202	High blood pressure	29.11%
1082	High cholesterol	26.20%
1452	Joint pain	35.17%
295	Migraines	7.14%
1099	Sleeping issues	26.62%
171	Thyroid problems	4.14%
455	Other	11.02%
761	No Answer	18.43%
11043	Total	

Q16: What are the food addiction issues FA helps you to address?
Please mark all that apply.

2387	Bingeing	57.81%
1789	Body image obsession	43.33%
407	Bulimia	9.86%
1497	Compulsive dieting	36.26%
3045	Food cravings	73.75%
2863	Food obsession	69.34%
2716	Grazing or eating all day	65.78%
2677	Obesity	64.83%
573	Over-exercising	13.88%
3195	Overeating	77.38%
983	Restricting food intake	23.81%
410	Undereating	9.93%
131	Other	3.17%
22673	Total	

Outcome Research of Food Addiction Treatment

Outcome research on alumnae of addiction-model food treatment programs indicates that many of the most advanced in their disease and historically impossible to treat can be helped significantly if they are treated intensively as if they are food addicts. It is well known in medicine that if the treatment works, the diagnosis was sufficient. Medicine is a very pragmatic art as well as a science.

There are now only about a dozen treatment programs for food addiction with long histories of success, but there are rigorous outcome studies of three of these. One was the inpatient program at Glenbeigh Psychiatric Hospital of Tampa, Florida, which was forced to close its doors when health insurance companies stopped reimbursing for hospital-based food addiction treatment. Another is the MFM outpatient program in Iceland which is also the base for the International Food Addiction

Counselor Training (INFACT). The third is a residential workshop-based program which works all over the world,[216] also the home of the ACORN/ SHiFT professional training program.

Outcome Survey of MFM Patients

MFM, an outpatient center for food addiction treatment outside of Reykjavik, Iceland, established in 2006, developed independently out of a recovery process involving GreySheeters Anonymous.

In 2017, Dr. Olof Asta Olofdotter MA, RN, RM, PhD, Professor at Iceland University, conducted a survey of the patients in the MFM Program to date. Five hundred questionnaires were sent, 325 clients opened the mail, and 282 completed the questionnaire, an 86.7% response rate.

Description of Research Group

The descriptive results showed that the majority of participants were women (87%) between 30-60 years old, with an academic degree (60%), having had an eating and a weight problem from a young age. Binge eating was experienced by 94%, purging and vomiting by 20%. Dieting had started when in childhood, from 5-15 years of age or from 20-30 years of age, often in relation to pregnancy, with fasting and/or starving behaviors (65%) and over exercising (20%). Over half had made efforts and used more than 7-10 ways to diet and try to lose weight. Added to the food problems, different psycho- and socio-cultural experiences existed, such as other types of addiction (42%) experiences of abuse and trauma in life (68%) and mental diseases (50%).[217] The length of treatment at MFM ranged from three months to more than a year.

Major findings of the research: Over 60% had periods of abstinence of more than a month to several years; 37% reported stable abstinence of over a year up to the time of the survey, having lost weight and reported positive emotional and physical outcomes; 20% stopped treating themselves as food addicts immediately after leaving the program.[218]

Most of this group continued actively in Twelve Step programs. They said they had a much more positive view towards life than before they came to MFM. Over 70% had periods of abstinence of over a month and reported strong positive emotional results from the MFM program. The length of abstinence varied from 1-6 months (30%) to more than a year (30%). Ninety percent of the respondents lost weight; 50% lost 25-60 pounds; 17% lost more than that.

ACORN/SHiFT is an international organization established in 1996 to present lectures and experiential workshops to educate about food addiction recovery. The ACORN Primary Intensive© is a five-day residential workshop that simulates the first week of in-patient food addiction treatment. Participants receive an individualized food plan, a recovery workbook, and five basic lectures on food addiction. During the week, each member commits each meal to a peer sponsor and inventories any problems they have being abstinent physically, emotionally, mentally, and spiritually. All participants also have a daily reading and "First Step" writing assignment on the topic of their powerlessness over food. They conclude by developing a threefold aftercare program: (1) for the day they leave, (2) for a general week back at home, and (3) for 90 days to a year.[219]

Outcome research includes clinical evaluations of 1318 clients between 1994 and 2008. Of these, 71% said they were not abstinent before coming to the event, about 10% never having been rigorously abstinent at all.[220] Over 99% were rigorously abstinent physically by the end of the workshop, and the average weight loss for alumnae one year after the workshop was 51 pounds from their previous highest weight.[221] ACORN Primary Intensive key results found:

- 2/3 were not food abstinent before the intensive, and most were not able to maintain stable food abstinence; 99% experienced substantial physical detox and were rigorously abstinent by the end of the five-day residential workshop.

- After a year, most saw themselves as food addicted and needing to abstain completely from their binge foods:

  o 83% eliminated sugar

  o 79% weighed and measured

  o 68% eliminated flour

  o 68% eliminated alcohol

  o 51% eliminated at least one other food.

- After a year, 70% were working a program in Overeaters Anonymous, smaller percentages in GreySheeters Anonymous, Food Addicts Anonymous, Food Addicts in Recovery Anonymous, and Recovering Food Addicts Anonymous.

- 91% incorporated prayer and meditation.

In a 2006 survey, 256 alumnae[222] (who had attended workshops 3-5 years previously) completed an eight-page questionnaire. Most (95%) were self-assessed food addicts who were not abstinent when they first participated in an ACORN workshop. At the time of the survey, a large majority (76%) were food abstinent, with an average 50-pound weight loss from their highest weight. Abstinence is a much higher standard than simple weight loss or "making progress towards recovery of an eating disorder." Abstinence means that a person is not using chemically addictive foods at all and is able to commit specific foods daily and eat what they commit.

Glenbeigh Hospital of Tampa Residential Treatment Program

The residential food addiction treatment program of Glenbeigh Psychiatric Hospital of Tampa was a six- to eight-week program for anorexics, bulimics, and overweight people who met the diagnostic criteria of a substance use disorder regarding food. They often had co-diagnoses of other addictions, such as alcoholism or drug addiction, and psychiatric diagnoses of depression, anxiety, and bipolar disorder.

The goal of the program was complete detoxification from addictive substances, developing an understanding of addictive diseases, and being prepared to do longer-term recovery after treatment, usually in food-related Twelve Step programs.

The program was designed to adapt the addiction model for alcoholism and drug addiction to food addiction. There were two days of multidisciplinary assessments. Patients were given a food plan that eliminated sugar, flour, excess fat, alcohol, and other personal binge foods. Patients committed their food daily to a peer sponsor, weighed and measured each meal, and practiced sharing honestly about the experience in a process group. There were daily lectures on the addictive concept of food addiction, a family week, and progressive assignments towards a full descriptive account of the patient's history regarding powerlessness over food. This writing work was repeated until counselors and the peer community were convinced that the patients had an in-depth grasp of their powerlessness over food addiction. The program included daily work on developing personal emotional skills to express and deal with difficult feelings. Aftercare programs included a local sponsor and usually ninety OA-HOW meetings in 90 days.

In 1993, Mary Theodora Carroll completed her PhD dissertation evaluating 71 female bulimic binge-purgers, bulimic binge eaters, and non-bulimic obese one to four years post-treatment to assess success rates. Over 2/3 of the sample group were food addiction abstinent at the time of the survey, half of the 2/3 being continuously abstinent every day since treatment. All those who were abstinent were stably at a healthy weight or moving towards it.[223]

This evaluation of food addiction treatment indicates conclusively that even the most difficult cases of food as a substance use disorder can be effectively treated. The patients at Glenbeigh Hospital of Tampa were late- and final-stage food addicts. Most of the patients had: 1) tried several diets, usually losing weight and regaining it; 2) had been in therapy using an eating-disorder model; and 3) had tried seriously to work an Overeaters Anonymous Twelve Step program and were unable to be abstinent or relapsed. The levels of multi-year abstinence from food addiction were comparable to the length of sobriety in the best residential treatment programs for alcoholism and other drug addictions.

Food Addiction Recovery for Young People

Two promising programs suggest that the food addiction recovery model may be effective regarding childhood obesity.

Dr. Robert Pretlow, a pediatric physician, developed a website to enable obese children to share their stories and communicate with each other about their issues with food. He collected 134,000 messages on his open-access interactive website www.weigh2rock.com. When he analyzed the children's own words, he found that the foods with which the kids had the most problem were the commonly addictive foods. When the kids tried to eliminate these foods completely, they experienced a period of withdrawal, after which cravings and obsessions were minimized or went away altogether. Most children had the characteristics of a substance use disorder, according to the DSM-4 criteria of the American Psychiatric Association. Dr. Pretlow has been designing weight loss programs which incorporate substance dependence treatment methods, i.e., addiction medicine.[224]

Another promising program is the previously-mentioned sugar-free program at Browns Hill Elementary and Magnet School in Lithonia GA, just outside Atlanta. The Principal, Dr. Yvonne Sanders-Butler, convinced the Board, the PTA, the teachers, and the students to create a sugar-free zone in and around the school. Sweetened beverages and snacks were removed from the vending machines. The school cafeteria eliminated added sugars from the lunch menu. Parents agreed to make similar diets available to the children. Children with their parents' support asked the stores on the way to school to put junk food in the back, rather than at the front of the store. In her book *Healthy Kids, Smart Kids,* Dr. Sanders-Butler presents evidence that children in the sugar-free program became healthier, their grades and standardized test scores improved, and truancy and behavior problems were reduced.[225]

FOOD ADDICTION DENIAL
NO. 8

Denial Statement #8: "No one ever robbed a bank to buy sugar or junk food; the personal and social consequences for food addiction are not as serious as they are for alcoholism or other drug addictions."

Rebuttal: First, food addicts do not rob banks because junk food is much less expensive than alcohol and not illegal. However, most of those who become food addicted at an early age have snuck (stolen) food from their parents or stores, and many have stolen money from their parents (their family bankers) to buy sweets and junk food. Second, the negative personal consequences for food addicts can be quite bad, and the social consequences of obesity and eating disorders (as much as half caused by food addiction) are devastating to the national health system. Third, it is arguable that as many die of food addiction as of drug addiction each year; they just use longer and die later. Some critical-stage alcoholics and drug addicts were first addicted to sugar, an "entry" drug biochemically.

CHAPTER 8

NEGATIVE CONSEQUENCES

"No one ever robbed a bank to buy food?"

Unless you work with late-stage food addicts extensively, you probably don't know that the vast majority of them stole food when they were young, stole money to buy food, then lied about it. This is not the same as stealing money to buy drugs, but it is close.

First, we are not talking about the child who snuck a taste of the dessert before dinner. We are talking about a young child who steals regularly, sometimes daily.

Second, it may not seem egregious for children to sneak food from their family's kitchen, but where else are they going to get at food when they cannot go out of the house alone?

Third, taking pennies, nickels, and dimes off their parents' bed stand may not be on the same scale as an adult robbing a bank or gas station, but who is the bank for a young child? Further, what if the change is consistently used to sneak out of the house or to a corner store on the way to school to buy candy, ice cream, or soda?

Fourth, food is cheap compared to alcohol and drugs, and it's legal, so just a handful of coins will buy enough sweets for a serious binge.

To take this story a little further, when recovering food addicts tell their secrets in treatment, they are clear that the early sneaking, stealing, and lying about food was against their values, and many escalate the lying as they get older. When challenged to do it for their own recovery, it is common for food addicts to self-disclose a wide range of theft for food:

- Bargaining for or stealing the desserts in other kids' school lunches.

- Trying to get extra treats at school.

- Hovering around the candy bowl at social gathering.

- Taking binge foods off the shelves in grocery stores, sometimes even when parents are with them.

- Raiding the refrigerator and cupboards at others' homes while babysitting.

The list goes on. While not all childhood food addicts do all of these and some do very few, many are quite manipulative in getting hold of their stash.

This leads to a theory which has not yet been researched but is interesting to consider. Is it possible that sugar and other commonly addictive food substances are gateway drugs for addictive substances we commonly consider more dangerous?

Science has a similar theory—with a lot of empirical evidence— that once a person's brain has been chemical altered to a critical level by an addictive substance, when the person completely eliminates the substance to recover, the brain unconsciously seeks out a replacement.[226] In the area of food addiction, for example, we find that a significant minority of bariatric surgery patients who follow the doctor's orders to minimize added sugar become clinically addicted to alcohol or other drugs of abuse within a year or two—even if they had no problems with alcohol or drugs prior to surgery.[227] Food addiction treatment professionals observe that many patients have a long history of switching back and forth between food bingeing and out-of-control shopping, codependent relationships, or sex.[228] Scientifically, this problem is called "kindling"; one addictive substance makes the brain more receptive and sometimes in serious need of an alternative.[229] In counseling, therapists often speak of healthy intimate relationships as being a recovery substitute. The Twelve Step solution is to build an individual spiritual practice which develops a healthy interdependency with God, or as they say,[230] "God as you understand God." There are innumerable other spiritual or religious paths.

Early stealing and lying about manipulating to get addictive foods frequently leads to a wide range of other self-centered behaviors in which food addicts manipulate not just for food, but also in other ways. Here are a few rather unique examples which show how close food addiction can parallel the development of alcoholism.

- In Maine, a compulsive overeater was pulled over for "driving while eating." He was swerving back and forth from lane to lane, pulled over by the police, put in jail for the night, and given a DUI (with no evidence of drinking).

- A woman pulled into a fast-food store, went in, and bought double hamburgers, large fries, and cokes (for herself). When she came out, she started eating so furiously that she forgot to strap her child into her car seat, pulled out into traffic, and was almost hit by another car. Her child fell off the seat and, fortunately, was not seriously hurt.

- An older man was eating out of a bag of groceries he had just bought. He got to a coffee cake just as he was going over a bridge. When he reached down into the bag for the coffee cake, he had trouble grabbing it and swerved the car toward the bridge's guardrail. Although the car teetered on the guardrail, he insisted on getting the coffee cake before he was willing to get out of the car.

- A woman was overeating in a restaurant with her binge buddies. She was especially looking forward to an ice cream sundae which she had the waiter bring with the rest of her meal. Towards the end of the meal, she looked down, and the dessert was missing. She accused her friends of taking it, but they—quite seriously—said that she had eaten it herself. She had completely blacked out the experience.

Some may judge these food addiction treatment stories as outlandish, even fanciful; but they are just more dramatic examples of stories told as recovering food addicts are in a place where they find honesty valued and encouraged.[231]

There is more quantitative research, such as the study that found soda causes 184,000 deaths per year worldwide, 25,000 in the United States alone,[232] and the conclusion that more people die of obesity each year than of opioid addiction.[233]

Let's look at the negative personal and social consequences of food addiction more analytically.

Negative Personal Consequences

It's not fun to be fat or to be bingeing and purging over the toilet frequently, but this is the day-to-day experience of most moderate-level food addicts. Other irritating experiences include: constant chafing between the thighs, not being able to fit in an airplane seat, being exhausted after climbing a set of stairs, breaking chairs in someone else's house, being caught taking someone else's food, and lying about all of the above. A majority of food addicts do their eating in private (ashamed of what others might see) and seldom disclose their most painful experiences. Here is one early-stage case study.

Case Study: Carla

Carla was a young Puerto Rican lawyer. She had been an excellent student and now was a prize find at a small prestigious New York law firm. Her boss said that he found her attractive, but he wished that she would lose about 25 pounds. She tried, but every diet ended the same; after some quick weight loss, the pounds came back on. At first, Carla wrote off the problem to stress cause by her case load, to being the only minority, and to constantly having to push back at the flirting of her boss without getting him too mad.

When she was interviewing another young woman lawyer for the firm, they talked a bit about their mutual weight problem, and Carla learned about GreySheeters Anonymous. She went to a few meetings and found that she actually liked the food plan: no sugar, no grain and no alcohol. Without even getting a sponsor or working the rest of the program, Carla started to lose weight, and this time she kept it off as long as she didn't deviate from the food plan. She started to have more energy and feel better about herself. Paradoxically, as she started feeling more attractive, Carla was able to confront her boss both about his fatism and his sexism. She considered it a quiet victory.

Carla learned enough about food addiction and was at an early stage such that she did not need the ongoing support of the program, or even to work the full program while she attended meetings.

Here is a case from the other end of the spectrum, a person in a very late or final stage who needed more than either a Twelve Step program or a so-called residential "food addiction" program could provide.

Case Study: Charlottie

Charlottie was an older African American woman who lived almost entirely confined to her home because it was difficult for her to get out of the front door. She need a pickup truck—and help to get in and out—to travel any distance. She was well over 400 pounds, but it had been a long time since she found a scale on which she could be weighed.

She had gained all this weight in the last twenty years, and Charlottie was puzzle by this because when she was married and younger, she and her husband developed a serious problem with alcohol. Her husband said he didn't want to quit, and Charlottie divorced him. Charlottie immediately stopped drinking "cold turkey," and she hadn't had a drop of alcohol since the day of her divorce. Why, she kept wondering, could she not just stop eating all the extra food as she had stopped the alcohol?

Charlottie now lived with her younger daughter, who cooked and helped around the house. The daughter also tried to help Charlottie with her diet, though the young girl was overweight, too. One day, the daughter was reading about Overeaters Anonymous and decided to attend a meeting (for her mother). After the meeting, she talked with members about how her mother was housebound. The group members offered to bring a meeting to Charlottie's home.

This worked out really well for several months. Charlottie liked the meetings and liked the spiritual program, but it seemed that she was not losing any weight. A bit of investigation found that her daughter had decided that it was unfair to deprive her mother of her favorite foods (even though they were not on the food plan), and Charlottie felt "obliged" to eat what her daughter prepared—and have seconds when they were offered. Talking to the daughter did not help. She did not believe sugar was dangerous at all (she ate it herself all the time).

This effort faded, but Charlottie's persistence got her into a residential program which prepared people for having weight loss surgery. She needed to lose at least 150 pounds, they said, for the surgery to be safe. The program advertised itself as being a "food addiction treatment"; but as it turned out, every patent had a phone, and they could order food from the outside. Charlottie joined her roommate in ordering two large pizzas every day. (Needless to say, this did not support her obtaining the needed weight loss.)

Without revealing the name of the program, this shows that, however well intended, professional food addition treatment at this center was in name only. Charlottie became more and more desperate, as she had still not found the support she needed and the support she was willing to accept. Her life was really not much better than that of an untreated late-stage alcoholic.

The negative personal consequences of the middle- and late-stage food addict can be in the range of failures in their lives caused by their progressive powerlessness over food. As stated in the *Twelve Steps and Twelve Traditions of Overeaters Anonymous*:

When we look with complete honesty at our lives, we see that where eating is concerned, we have acted in an extremely irrational and self-destructive manner. Under the compulsion to overeat, many of us have done things no sane person would think of doing. We have driven miles in the dead of night to satisfy a craving for food. We have eaten food that was frozen, burnt, stale, or even dangerously spoiled. We have eaten food off of other people's plates, off the floor, off the ground. We have dug food out of the garbage and eaten it.

We have frequently lied about what we have eaten – lied to others because we didn't want to face the truth ourselves. We have stolen food from our friends, family, and employers, as well as from the grocery store. We have also stolen money to buy food. We have eaten beyond the point of being full, beyond the point of being sick of eating. We have continued to overeat, knowing all the while we were disfiguring and maiming our bodies. We have isolated ourselves to eat, damaging our relationships and denying ourselves a full social life. For the sake of our compulsive eating, we have turned ourselves into objects of ridicule, and we have destroyed our health.

Then, horrified by what we were doing to ourselves with food, we became obsessed with diets. We spent hundreds of dollars on weight-loss schemes, we bought all sorts of appetite-control drugs, we joined nightclubs and bars, we had ourselves hypnotized and analyzed, we had major surgery on our digestive systems, we had our ears stapled or our jaws wired shut. All of this we did willingly, hoping we could someday "have our cake and eat it too. "

Some of us went from doctor to doctor looking for a cure. The doctors gave us diets, but we had no better success with those than with the other diets we'd been on. The doctors gave us shots and pills. Those worked for a while, but we inevitably lost control and overate again, putting back on the weight we had worked so hard to lose.

Many of us tried fasting, with and without a doctor's supervision. Usually we lost weight, but as soon as we started eating again, the compulsive eating behavior returned, along with the weight. Some of us learned to purge ourselves with vomiting, laxatives, or excessive exercise. We'd stuff food in our mouths until we were in physical pain, then we'd "get rid of it." We damaged our digestive system and our teeth while we starved our bodies of nutrients needed to live.

Those of us who are overweight got plenty of advice from others about how to get our "ideal "size, but nothing permanently solved our problem. We found that no matter what we did to ease our turmoil, our compulsive eating eventually returned. Over the long haul, our weight went up and our self-esteem went down. After a while we became battle-weary and discouraged. Still, we could never accept our powerlessness. The prospect of being obese, sick, and out of control for the rest of our lives led some of us to conclude that life was simply not worth living. Many of us thought about suicide. Some of us tried it.

Most of us, however, never reached suicidal desperation. Instead, we took comfort in a feeling that everything was all right as long as we got enough to eat.

Instead of bringing comfort, the overeating backfired. The more we ate the more we suffered, yet we continued to overeat. Our true insanity could be seen in the fact that we kept right on trying to find comfort in excess food, long after it began to cause us misery.

Once we honestly looked at our lives, it became easy for us to admit we had acted insanely where food and weight were concerned. Many of us, however, were able to confine our compulsive eating to the hours when we were alone and to carry on with relatively normal lives. We worked hard during the day and ate hard at night. Surely we were sane in most respects.[234]

Not all food addicts have all of these problems, but many of these issues are familiar to most food addicts who have still not found and accepted the solution.

Negative Medical Consequences of Food Addiction

In Nancy Appleton's *Lick the Sugar Habit,* she discusses how sugar addiction upsets the whole body chemistry. It is already well known that the obese are more prone to diabetes, heart disease, depression, back and joint problems, respiratory disorders, and some forms of cancer.[235] Appleton provides examples of several degenerative diseases and harmful conditions suffered by food addicts: "hypoglycemia, hyperglycemia, constipation, intestinal gas, asthma, headaches, psoriasis, arthritis, premenstrual syndrome, candidiasis, obesity, osteoporosis, tooth decay, multiple sclerosis, inflammatory bowel disease, chancre sores, gallstones, kidney stones, cystic fibrosis."[236]

There are also secondary medical dangers for those with bulimia: "decay of tooth enamel, electrolyte imbalance, anxiety and panic attacks, dark circles and puffiness under the eyes, obsession with food and weight and body shape, isolation from family, hyperactivity, swollen glands under the jaw, personality changes—from outgoing to withdrawn, memory failure, dangerous rapid heartbeat, lightheadedness, and suicide."[237]

Here is a case study of a typical bulimic food addict.

Case Study: Lily

Lily grew up in a suburban home with parents who were moving from lower to middle class. A lot of emphasis was placed on achievement, and Lily was fairly successful throughout her academic career.

During puberty, Lily had some stress regarding her body, thinking that her new "curves" were really fat. She got over this mainly by discussing it openly with her peers.

When she went to college, Lily gained the "freshman fifteen pounds" but took the weight off by restricting calories. Her sophomore year, she joined a sorority, and there she learned the trick of "eating your food and having your figure, too." The trick was purging after overeating.

After college, most of Lily's sorority sisters stopped overeating so they could stop purging. They didn't like "heads in the toilet." However, Lily was obsessed with food and didn't want to cut back on her favorites. If anything, now that she had a decent-paying job, why couldn't she eat what she wanted? So Lily increased her purging.

She went from one binge and one purge each evening to bingeing and purging at lunch and dinner. Then she added extra evening eating and purging. She became concerned when she recognized that she was overeating and purging more often, and she went to an eating disorder therapist.

Lily enjoyed counseling. It was a relief to tell someone her "secret." She began to consider that if she dealt with her underlying issues, she might not have to binge and purge at all anymore. Lily felt satisfied with the insights regarding her youth and family life that therapy afforded. After about a year, however, she was still binging and purging, almost as much as before. Her therapist suggested Food Addicts in Recovery Anonymous (FA).

The idea that she might be overeating because she had become chemically dependent on sugar and flour, like alcoholics and drug addicts become dependent on their drug of choice, was a revelation. Even more amazing to Lily was that when she committed her food to another recovering food addict and committed not to purge one day at a time, she was able to do that. She joined a special AWOL group to work on the Twelve Steps, found this even more life enhancing, and accepted the FA program as her new way of life.

Here is a more complex case of an anorexic and bulimic food addict whose disease was more progressed.

Case Study: Meghan

Meghan came from a very turbulent family and was tall for her age. She developed a biting sense of humor as her major coping skill to deal with her family and in her social life. She did well in school and played a number of sports. She was especially good in basketball and volleyball and obtained a college scholarship for the latter.

From the beginning, Meghan had problems with the college volleyball coach. He wanted her to lose weight. Almost as a reaction, she thought, she gained weight. When this threatened her place on the team, she did what other girls were doing—she started to restrict her food intake between binges and then, when this didn't work, she began to purge by vomiting. Meghan was quite open about this with her peers, as it was not unusual on the volleyball team.

Her junior year, Meghan started to fast for more than one day at a time. One day, she fainted on the volleyball court. She was sent to the school doctor, who decided her eating disorder was severe enough that she needed to go to treatment. She was in residential treatment for six weeks, declared cured, and returned to school in time for the volleyball season.

Within a few weeks, Meghan was back to arguing with the coach and bingeing and purging.

Her senior year, Meghan told her counselor that she needed to return to treatment. Again, she was very successful in all aspects of treatment, but it was recommended that she stop playing volleyball. When she did stop, she also decided to drop out of school. Her counselor told her there was something wrong in her thinking, but Meghan was stubborn. She returned during the summer to complete her last classes and graduate.

At this point, Meghan decided that she was never going to binge or purge again. Periodic fasting was OK. For eight years, she kept to her commitment. During this time, she developed a career as nanny, got married, and had a child.

Then one day Meghan had the thought, "it would be safe to have just one binge"; and when she did, she also rationalized purging. It was downhill from there. Within a few months, she was bingeing and purging at almost every meal, finding excuses to go outside and purge in the bushes so her daughter couldn't see. She decided to return to eating disorder treatment.

This time, the treatment did not work as well. Meghan found herself sneaking sugar/flour products and eating them on the sly during her treatment. When she started purging, one of the staff smelled it on her breath, and she was asked to leave. She felt hopeless.

Back at work, the mother for whom Meghan worked told her about food addiction and a treatment program that had helped her when she was younger. This began a series of short visits to food addiction treatment programs, where she learned to be abstinent from her binge foods and use a Twelve Step program for support. She also continued her work on unresolved trauma from her anorexia and bulimia. Megan now started to have periods for about a year at a time when she was abstinent and felt positive about herself. She still needed periodic recharges, and still does.

It is not surprising that those with obesity are likely to have an average five-year shortened lifespan.[238] It is not yet clear what percentage of those with obesity and bulimia are food addicted, nor whether health problems are more or less if you are food addicted than if you are not. However, the almost universal effects for those who are food addicted are weight gain or inappropriate weight loss, severe weight gain, depression, low self-image, and loss of spirit.

Negative Social Consequences

A major social cost of food addiction is the expense of health care. Obesity is one of the biggest drivers of preventable chronic disease and healthcare cost in the United States.[239] Food addiction is one of the biggest drivers of obesity.[240] In 2012, the cost of obesity was estimated to range from $147 billion to nearly $210 billion per year.[241] If one third of the obese are food addicted, a modest estimate, then the cost of food addiction is $50-$70 billion a year.[242] In addition, obesity is associated with job absenteeism, costing approximately $4.3 billion annually[243] and with lower productivity while at work, costing employers $506 per obese worker per year.[244]

Healthcare costs go up with increases in BMI. Obese people's healthcare costs are 28% more than overweight people, and severely obese people's healthcare costs are 41% more than overweight people.[245] Similarly, according to the American Heart Association, as a person's BMI increases, so do the average number of sick days, medical claims, and healthcare costs.[246] According to the Trust for America's Health, Medicare could save more than $5 billion, and Medicaid could save more than $1.9 billion by expanding the use of prevention programs regarding obesity.[247] No distinction was made between obesity caused by food addiction and obesity developed from other causes, but it can be assumed that a percentage of these significant cost savings could be obtained from appropriate food addiction prevention and treatment.

In summary, the social costs of food addiction are substantial. While alcohol and drugs are considerably more expensive than addictive foods, and abuse of food is not illegal, the pain cost to individuals and the health costs of food addiction nationally are comparable to those of alcoholism and drug addiction. Put another way, if food addiction and obesity are not brought under control, just the ongoing medical costs for care of chronic diseases such as diabetes could break the medical system in the United States.

FOOD ADDICTION DENIAL
NO. 9

Denial Statement #9: "Bariatric surgery is the only effective treatment for obesity."

Rebuttal: Surgery can be productive for many of the obese who are in critical health situations and need extraordinary medical intervention. However, bariatric surgery usually does not work for those with advanced food addiction. There is evidence that another extraordinary intervention, food addiction treatment, can be helpful for many who relapse after surgery.

CHAPTER 9

LIMITS OF BARIATRIC SURGERY

In 2009, a middle-aged woman was sitting in the office of her bariatric surgeon, crying out of control. She had had successful surgery about a year before, but then could not stop eating. She very quickly learned that she could eat a pint of ice cream at a time and get it to stay down. As soon as there was room for more, she went out and bought more ice cream. She had gone to her surgeon several times. He had suggested tips that often worked for others; they didn't work for her. He recommended a therapist, but this did not help, either. By now, she was actually eating more. We met the surgeon at a workshop and said, "We understand."

It turns out that his patient might have been one of the many examples of bariatric surgery patients unable to lose weight in spite of the surgery.[248] An unpublished survey of bariatric surgeons that year found that 15-20% of their clients either did not lose weight or regained most of their weight within the first year.[249]

At the same time, we were learning, one case at a time, that an intensive workshop for food addiction recovery worked as well for those having unsuccessful surgeries as it did for binge eating and bulimic food addicts who had not had the surgery.

Case Study: Norma

Norma was a Washington lawyer who was very successful in her field but unable to apply the same discipline and willpower to losing excess weight or maintaining a healthy weight. Over a ten-year period, she lost and regained over fifty pounds four times. She was now close to that "never again" weight of 300 pounds. She applied and was accepted for bariatric surgery. The surgery was successful, and she lost over 100 pounds during the first year. Then "it started happening again." By the end of the second year, Norma was within twenty pounds of her previously highest weight.

Norma tried Overeaters Anonymous, but she was unable to develop a stable abstinence with a sponsor. She heard of a five-day residential workshop program that had helped many other OAs. She went. At the workshop, she was given a food plan containing no flour or sugar or any of her other binge foods. She went through some symptoms of withdrawal—fatigue, irritability, and strong cravings—but they went away after three days, and she was rigorously abstinent by the end of the workshop. Norma did some emotional work regarding feelings of fear and anger which arose when she was abstinent. She also listened to four lectures on food addiction recovery and worked on a number of assignments to describe specific times when she was powerless over food. She was helped to develop an aftercare plan and returned home successfully working an Overeaters Anonymous program.

Two years later, Norma was unable to get out of a depression with the help of her therapist and began using sugar and flour products again. She returned to the food addiction workshop, became abstinent again, and has remained so eight years later.[250]

There are now dozens of such cases. Some are less complicated, and some are more complex and take longer to resolve.

Ten years ago, members of Overeaters Anonymous who had had bariatric surgery often did not disclose this information in meetings or even to their sponsors. They considered it shameful to have gone to such great lengths and still be unable to control their eating or their weight. Today, it is common for members of OA and of the other food-related Twelve Step fellowships to share that surgery was one of their experiments that did not work. Many find it possible to put down the food and achieve stable weight loss just by using the OA or Food Addicts in Recovery (FA) programs.

One much more advanced case is that of a younger woman who had three separate bariatric surgeries, the second two because the prior surgeries had not produced successful results. Unfortunately, she was also one of the food addicts for whom a single week-long residential workshop was insufficient, and she was unwilling to participate in more workshops or to go to longer residential food addiction treatment. One characteristic common among food addicts was that she wanted a "quick fix," and she wanted a food addiction recovery program which included eating her "favorite foods."[251]

There are several cases of people with late- or final-stage food addiction who were willing to do for their food recovery what many late-stage alcoholics and drug addicts must do for theirs.

Case Study: Summer

Summer was a Master's level mental health therapist who was especially skilled at developing peer support groups. Thus, she felt especially guilty and ashamed that she was unable to follow her own guidance when she went to Weight Watchers. She worked the program, but never successfully for more than two or three days at a time. She went to Food Addicts Anonymous (FAA) and had similar problems. She worked with several different sponsors, tried to use all the tools of the program, and worked through the Steps with guidance. Within a couple of months, she was back eating and was spending all of her disposable income on food.

She came to us asking whether we thought it was a good idea for her to go to residential treatment for food addiction. It was a stretch economically, and her parents, who were retired, were reluctant to pay. We suggested that she go to treatment, and her parents decided to help out. After four weeks, Summer was stably abstinent but really afraid that she was not going to keep this up when she went back to the world outside of treatment.

Summer negotiated a plan where she would assist in cooking at our five-day workshops in return for being able to sit in on groups. This was unusual, but we saw her as particularly motivated. With this extra support on a regular basis, Summer slowly moved towards a stable abstinence. At first, she needed to do a "recovery job" outside her field at Wal-Mart; but a year or so later, she was able to return to working in her field.[252]

Exploratory research at a bariatric surgery program in Massachusetts found that about a fifth of those patients already cleared for surgery, but not having surgery yet, assessed themselves as being addicted to specific foods. It may not be a coincidence that a similar percentage of those completing surgery present with characteristics of food as a substance use disorder, physical craving and loss of control, as well as significant weight gain or difficulty losing weight. In this same study, three fifths of the prospective bariatric surgery patients assessed themselves as "emotional eaters." It is worth noting that in treatment, many who turned out to be food addicts started by saying that they were or wanted to be people with eating disorder problems, i.e., psychologically-based issues.[253]

Also, many bariatric surgery practices have been discovering that one or two years after surgery, a significant number of their patients become seriously addicted to alcohol or drugs. One study found that 10-15% became what I would call "cross-addicted." In these cases, patient histories found that they had no prior problems with alcohol or drugs at a clinical level, so the alcoholism or drug addiction was not a matter of relapse. Rather, these were likely patients who followed doctor's advice and avoided or moderated the use of sugar, and then the addictive part of their brain found another substance of abuse. More research on this is needed, but there is no theory that seems more persuasive at this time.[254]

More recently, in the latest textbook of Food Addicts in Recovery Anonymous, Dr. Carl Lowe Jr. is cited both for his diagnosis of many of his patients as being food addicted as well as for a practical way of integrating Twelve Step food addiction support into his surgery practice.

As quoted by Dr. Lowe in *Food Addicts in Recovery Anonymous*,

This is exactly what my patients need.

Most bariatric surgeons hold support groups at least monthly, but a meeting once a month or even once a week is not enough to help a person deal with the day-to-day yearnings and cravings to eat certain foods. I loved FA. Each of the members had a sponsor, someone he or she could talk with daily. The people there were the warmest you could ever meet, and the results were amazing. I saw people who had lost 60 pounds and 100 pounds. I even met a woman who had lost 200 pounds.

FA seemed to me to be a perfect solution. It offered wonderful support, frequent meetings, and a human being who could talk with a struggling person every single day until he or she got strong.

The clincher for me is the spiritual nature of the program. We are all humans. We all have frailties. We don't have the strength and the power to do many of the things in life that we think we can do. When you are in a situation of addiction and you start believing that you can pull yourself up by your bootstraps and solve the problem yourself, you are destined for failure. Clearly, the addiction has the upper hand. That's what makes it an addiction—it's something that you cannot control.

In addiction, you are facing a spiritual battle, a psychological and physical battle. You have to have a partner right with you. You cannot do it by yourself. You need other people and you need a higher power. Until and unless you acknowledge that fact and allow a higher power to come into your life, you are doomed. Twelve-step programs like Food Addicts in Recovery Anonymous and Alcoholics

Anonymous, which are based on spiritual recovery, have long track records of success. Why fight what works so well?[255]

There are also significant examples of integrating assessment and treatment of food addiction related to bariatric surgery from the experience of a professional food addiction therapist. In Werdell's *Bariatric Surgery and Food Addiction: Preoperative Considerations,* there are three case studies, one of a food addict who was assessed and treated prior to bariatric surgery, one of a recovered alcoholic who used food-related Twelve Step support after bariatric surgery, and one of a surgery patient who, after losing a great deal of weight and then regaining it all and more, used food addiction treatment as a successful alternative.

Case Study: Maria

Maria, a 5'5" 334-lb. opera singer, had been a member of OA-HOW for just over 30 days when we met. More than a year later, she had lost 90 pounds and was uncertain about having bariatric surgery. I told her I was writing a book on the topic and asked her to write her story as she had told me.

She wrote that she had struggled with her weight for ten years before investigating the surgery. After two years, she was well into the process because her weight had begun causing serious health issues. At one point, it struck her that her problem might be more than physical. As her father had been an advanced alcoholic, Maria suspected that she might also be an addict, with food as her drug of choice. On June 23, 2007, Maria had found herself awake in front of her refrigerator but had no idea how she had gotten there. Since her father had suffered from blackouts, she considered that blackouts might also be responsible for her weight gain. She googled "food addiction," and it led her to OA.

The OA program worked for Maria; she thanks God for OA, which helped her lose weight and keep it off longer than she had ever been able to do so previously.[256]

Case Study: Jim

Jim was a long-time recovered alcoholic who shifted from alcohol to food and tried Overeaters Anonymous but couldn't put the food down. He dropped out of OA because for him, "it didn't work." Finally, at his doctor's urging, he became a candidate for bariatric surgery, took weekly classes for six months, lost 20 pounds, was accepted, and had the surgery as an outpatient. Bariatric surgery worked for Jim: A year later, he was 84 pounds below his top weight, with lab results in the healthy-normal range. He still attends an OA meeting weekly to keep the compulsion to overeat in check.[257]

Case Study: Deborah

Deborah had always considered herself a competent person—an Ivy League graduate with two degrees and one of the nation's first women ministers with her own congregation. The one area of life she could not control was her eating, or weight. After much yo-yo dieting, she tried OA but could never achieve a stable abstinence. At her doctor's urging, she elected bariatric surgery. At first, the surgery was a success—she lost more than 100 pounds, felt better, and had considerable improvement in her blood tests. Gradually, though, she began out-of-control overeating once again.

Someone referred Deborah to ACORN's five-day "Primary Intensive" for food addicts. Though she was skeptical, she decided to give it a try. By the end of the five days, she was "rigorously abstinent" from all her binge foods. After a few difficult days of detoxification, her food cravings had disappeared, and her "crazy thinking" about food had lessened incredibly.

Because she found she really wanted more structure and support, she returned to OA and has maintained a 220-pound weight loss, rigorously working her OA program daily.

Deborah views her failure after bariatric surgery as a positive. It helped her fully break her denial that she was food addicted, and it led her to a recovery program that works for her—physically, emotionally, and spiritually.[258]

These early cases of integrating bariatric surgery and food addiction treatment for obesity are promising. We have only initial reports from clinicians, so more rigorous research is needed.

In conclusion, bariatric surgery is not the correct answer for some overweight people who are also food addicts. Some food addicts are successful in recovery with intensive treatment for food addiction before or after their operation.

FOOD ADDICTION DENIAL
NO. 10

<u>Denial Statement #10</u>: "No one forces obese people to overeat; obviously, they are the ones who put the food in their mouths. Focusing on personal powerlessness over food is counterproductive; it brings a person down rather than increasing self-esteem."

<u>Rebuttal</u>: Normal Eaters do choose to eat; and if they overeat and gain weight, they can choose to diet and lose the weight. They are not powerless.

When a person is food addicted, someone else does not force the person to overeat; rather, it is the chemical dependency in their brain that overpowers their healthy thinking. They do become powerless. Food addiction is a disease, and no one would ever choose to have it—just like they would not choose to have diabetes, heart disease, or cancer. As physical cravings and mental obsessions get stronger, it becomes impossible for a food addict to fight them with reason and willpower alone. This is what we mean by addictive powerlessness.

One of the characteristics of addiction is being in denial that willpower alone can solve the problem. The disease itself fights against the idea that the food addict is powerless over food. When the denial is effectively challenged, food addicts see they are powerless alone over the disease, but they are not helpless. They can ask for and accept help from others; and if they believe in a spiritual higher power, they can invoke God as they understand God.

CHAPTER 10

POWERLESSNESS

Why the focus on identifying specific ways food addicts are powerless over food?

Food addiction, like alcoholism and all other addictions, is a brain disease: Specific foods create a biochemical change in the pleasure center and instinctive parts of the brain, making the food addict chemically dependent on the exact foods that progressively make the problem worse. Food addicts become powerless over these foods: They become powerless over physical cravings and powerless even over obsessive thoughts about these foods unless they abstain from the foods completely. If they break abstinence from their trigger foods, there will be times when they won't be able to tell the difference between physically addictive cravings and healthy hunger. Sometimes, once they start eating these foods, they won't be able to stop. In later stages of the disease, even when they are abstinent from these foods, mental obsessions will sometimes call them to start eating the dangerous foods.[259] Progressively, they are unable to differentiate between this addictive thinking and the healthy thinking that would stop them from starting to eat addictively again.

The three levels of powerlessness in food addiction are: physical craving, mental obsession, and addictive personality.[260]

I. Physical Craving

In early stages of the disease, it is necessary for food addicts to identify the foods that are toxic to them. Some need to do this repetitively because the cravings keep fooling them. Physical cravings are distorted hunger instincts in which a food addict doesn't just "need to eat," but rather, feels he or she "_has to eat._" For food addicts, physical cravings are a mental disorder. Food addicts have a sense of false starving; they think life is not worth living without certain foods or they have a thought like, "I'll die if I can't get this food." The only way to eliminate cravings is to eliminate the specific addictive foods entirely.[261]

In early recovery, developing an abstinent food plan is often a matter of trial and error. Many are surprised that they cannot do this by themselves and develop a plan that works for an extended period of time. It is common for food addicts to blame the source of their food plan—if they got the plan from a dietician, they will say the dietician is no good; if they got the food plan from a Twelve Step program, they will say Twelve Step programs don't work; or if they devised the food plan themselves, they will feel guilty or ashamed, especially if they have a long history of failure in dieting. An alternative explanation is that they are becoming powerless over the physical cravings seeping out of the addictive part of their minds. They are no more able to control these cravings by reason or willpower than are dyslexics able to control the way their minds mix up words or than a claustrophobic would be able to control being afraid in a closed elevator. Food addicts are as powerless over sugar cravings as drug addicts are powerless over cravings for cocaine, heroin, or oxycontin. The only way to eliminate food cravings is to eliminate the offending food to the extent that it causes craving, often completely.

Some food addicts do not see themselves as powerless until they notice how difficult it is to tell the truth to someone else about their food. When food addicts see and accept their powerlessness over cravings, they can pursue both the committing of their food to someone beyond themselves and rigorous honesty about any ways they do not completely honor this commitment as spiritual practice. This is often quite difficult. Recommitting to eliminate any foods that are problematic creates a habit of mind. For those who cannot do this alone, it makes sense to do this practice with another person—a therapist, a Twelve Step sponsor, or a friend who understands food addiction. For those who are consciously spiritual, this food commitment can be seen as a spiritual practice. Self-disclosure about any mistakes becomes part of this spiritual practice. There is a more in-depth discussion of inventorying food slips in my handbook by the same name.[263]

When recovering from food addiction, rigorous honesty often means being more specific. See the chart below about the progression from denial to rigorous honesty about being powerless.

Progression of Self Disclosure about a Break in Abstinence	
Level I: In Denial	I don't have a problem. It's going to be different. I'm not as bad as real food addicts. I should be able to be like other people. I can stop if I want to. I can deal with this by myself.
Level II: Admitting	I do have a problem. I'm different than a normal eater. I'm not as bad as some others yet. My way didn't work. I can't stop. I'm powerless—out of control. I need help.
Level III: Being Specific about the Food	I had a slip yesterday. I didn't eat exactly what I committed. I ate sugar. I binged on ice cream. I ate a whole pint of Haagen-Dazs Chocolate Chocolate Chip Ice Cream. I ate out of control with my fingers.
Level IV: Being specific about Feelings	Early that day, I decided to put down ice cream for good. I felt happy, committed, determined, a little excited … By the end of the day, I was shoveling down a pint of Haagen-Dazs with my fingers while I was driving. I felt frantic, crazed, and numb. I had a headache from eating so much cold ice cream so fast, but I couldn't stop. When it was gone, I wanted …
Level V: Being Specific about Being Powerless	… so when I went to throw it out, I had the thought, "Maybe I should save it in case I get a visitor who eats ice cream." It didn't feel like the best idea, but I said, "I can handle it." I went to work and had a good day, except that my boss didn't like a report I turned in at the end of the day. I as miffed, but didn't say anything. When I got home, I had the thought, "I'll just have a look at the ice cream in the freezer." I had a vague sense that this was not too good an idea, but I opened the freezer door anyway. Something subtly shifted inside me. I just stood there enjoying the coolness from the freezer coming at me. I was almost mesmerized by the picture of the ice cream in a dish on the package. The cravings became too powerful to resist. I had the thought, "Well, I could have just a little." I took the container out, opened it, and stuck my finger in it. It was very hard. I had to dig to get out a chunk, and I just crammed it into my mouth. It tasted sweet, delicious, but only for a moment. I swallowed the ice cream—it was still very cold and hard. There were flashes of negativity—"How could I do this again?" and feelings of guilt and shame, but I already had my fingers digging out more ice cream and thinking about finishing the whole pint before starting to eat the second bite. I felt crazed, out of control, like an animal.

©Phil Werdell, 2002

Food addicts in the early stages of the disease might have periods of control, might only eat a little more than they expected, might or might not develop a practice of total bingeing. The substantial periods of control at this stage are often an illusory proof to food addicts that they really are not powerless over their food intake.

II. Mental Obsession

In the middle stages of addiction, it is not uncommon for the disease to be more advanced. Besides physical cravings, most also developmental obsessions. The simple way of understanding the difference is this: cravings can make food addicts powerless to stop eating specific foods or large quantities of almost any foods once they have started; mental obsessions are the double whammy—mental obsessions can make food addicts powerless over beginning to eat the specific foods from which they need to abstain.

There is still more to learn scientifically about addictive thinking, but we *do* know that advanced food addicts are damaged in the cognitive and memory centers of their brains, just like the minds of alcoholics and drug addicts.[264] Mental obsessions, often called "stinking thinking" in the Twelve-Step rooms, are thoughts which are not true but which are believed to be true by the addictive mind.[265] The food addict will think:

- "I'll just have one,"
- "I *HAVE* to eat this!"
- "I'll start my diet tomorrow"
- "Others eat this with impunity,"
- "I just want this."
- "The hell with the rules."

They won't remember that in the past, they decided these thoughts— or dozens of other thoughts—were untrue. They won't remember the past negative consequences of overeating, or they will minimize them. In the present moment—and often for a long time—they are powerless to notice the irrationality of their food thoughts or to effectively resist acting on them. This is called "euphoric recall" and is common to all addictions.

From a practical point of view, my observation is that these mental obsessions arise specifically because the addictively damaged or chemically dependent part of the brain overpowers reason and the willpower to control eating. The damaged part of the brain overrides the healthy part of the brain by finding a particular thought or blank spot[266] that the food addict easily believes, EVEN THOUGH IT IS NOT TRUE AND ULTIMATELY DANGEROUS. Such thoughts actually increase in their believability—and often in their variety and number—as the disease progresses. It is this problem of powerlessness that any true food addiction recovery process must address.

This deeper understanding of powerlessness is something that must be taught through personal observation and feedback. Here are some examples:

- As addicts begin to understand physical craving and mental obsession more deeply, they might say, "I am powerless over donuts and the thoughts that 'I can just eat one,' or 'this time it won't matter.'" Or, more generally, they might say, "I am powerless over sugar and flour—and my thoughts about food that are addictive to me."

- One food addict found she frequently had a glass of wine before binging, and she always thought that "this time is different" or had just a mental blank spot about the many times this had ended badly in the past. Although she never binged on alcohol, she always binged on food after one drink. Finally, she said, "I am powerless over euphoric recall. "

- One very subtle example is the food addict who claimed, "I only binge on abstinent foods." This was a rationalization for eating extra foods on his food plan, but not sugar or flour. However, the principle upon which the food plan was built was "eliminating all binge foods." So the logical action would be to take the binge foods out of his food plan, rather than rationalizing he could eat them because they were on his food plan. Even though this issue was explained several times, the food addict "kept forgetting."[267]

Food addicts are oblivious to the fact that they rationalize their binging. Once they see that this has happened over and over again and that it is likely to continue happening, they can start saying with conviction, "I am powerless over my own thinking about food."

In active food addiction, the phenomenon of mental compulsion presents itself in endless ways. For those in relapse, especially chronic relapse, challenging this level of food addictive denial is an essential part of the work.

The Dishonesty-Honesty Continuum

Complete or Congenital Dishonesty	The text or "Big Book" of Alcoholics Anonymous calls this "constitutionally incapable of being honest." These are congenital liars who are *often not even aware that they are not telling the truth.*
Mean-Spirited Dishonesty	This is knowing that a lie will hurt someone and doing it anyway. This is intentional and malevolent dishonesty *even if being hurtful is just a part of the intention or a covert reason for the lie.*
Conscious Dishonesty	This is a bold-faced lie, consciously knowing what you are saying is not truthful. Such a lie is almost always selfish and self-centered, and there is usually the expectation that you will not get caught or, if you do, it will be worth the price.
Dishonesty by Omission	Often called a white lie, this is often done with the thought that you don't want someone else to get hurt. It is also the lie of the con person, showing attractive truth while hiding the deceptive underbelly.
Cash Register Honesty	This is telling the objective truth about objective matters. "You gave me too much change." "I did not eat the foods that I said I would." There is no indication of subjective reason or motivation
Tough Love Honesty	This is telling hard truths, often ones that the recipient might not want to hear, but being honest anyway with the intention of being helpful. This is not "brutal honesty" or saying whatever negative thoughts are on your mind regardless of the effect on others.
Rigorous Honesty	This is telling the complete truth, often about yourself, even though you are embarrassed or really do not want to reveal the information. It is being hard on yourself because this is the right thing to do – or because, if you are not this truthful, your abstinence is in danger.
Perfect Honesty	This is a level of honesty that is beyond the human capacity. It is the truth of God or of the spiritual realm unburdened by any human frailty. Though we may be instruments of this level of truth, we can never be perfectly certain that this is happening. As the book *Alcoholics Anonymous* puts it, "we are not saints."

For the food addict, there is no such thing as "perfect honesty," only "rigorous honesty" about everything, including their addictive thinking. Once food addicts have reached a critical level and understand their own powerlessness, they know they need help in discerning the truth from the false. Long-time food addicts develop a habit of checking out their own thinking about food. At first, they often work with a sponsor on a daily basis or with a therapist on a weekly basis to check out their food and recovery thinking. The therapist, sponsor, or sometimes a friend who understands food addiction serves as a "fair witness."

III. Addictive Personality

In the late and final stages of food addiction, there are even deeper levels of powerlessness. Sometimes advanced food addicts cannot even imagine what it would be like to live putting their food abstinence and recovery first in their lives. They see this as being "impractical" or "unrealistic," or they see themselves as being "hopeless" or "not having the willingness" to eliminate their binge foods completely or go to any length for their own health and spiritual recovery.[268]

This is the core of the disease, and every food addict has this problem to some degree: self-will run riot, selfishness and self-centeredness to an unhealthy point. However, like with late-stage alcoholics and other drug addicts, the highly progressed food addict needs to see, accept, and confront this problem directly.

This problem, often called the development of a false or addictive self, i.e., addictive personality,[269] is common in the food addicts we as professionals see. These are the people who could not on their own "just put down" the binge foods that were giving them so much trouble. Usually Cognitive Behavioral therapy (CBT) or traditional eating disorder talk therapy about underlying issues is not helpful in dealing with this level of chronic addictive thinking.

Many late-stage food addicts have even tried OA or other Twelve Step programs and been unable to achieve and maintain food abstinence and recovery. They found that just getting honest about being powerless over specific foods and specific addictive thoughts was insufficient.

The distortion in their personality is at the level of will and self-concept. Twerski, a noted addiction psychiatrist, says that the metal problems of an addict are much like those of a schizophrenic.[270] As mentioned previously, this is similar to what the AA text *Alcoholics Anonymous* says— that "the problem centers in the mind," and the addict is like Dr. Jekyll and Mr. Hyde.[271] Sometimes the food addict's consciousness is healthy and grounded in reality; other times, the addictive personality takes over.

A simple example of food-addicted personality is the 600-pound man in choir who questions over and over again why he "does this to himself" and responds, "I just like to eat." This man has not just rationalized overeating on specific occasions; he has rationalized overeating as a way of life. For most food addicts, the addictive personality is just a part of their consciousness. When the addictive personality completely overtakes food addicts, they do not even know that they are in denial.

Here is an example of a late-stage food addict describing how her life is almost always focused on food, what she can eat, or how she can diet.

Case Study: Ginger

Why I'm convinced I'm powerless over food:

- *After I do something, especially something difficult, I instantly think of eating "a treat"—the thought awakens me and brightens me up.*

- *When I hear of, or see, or think of a binge food, I instantly feel I must get it immediately.*

- *When I'm at an event where cake or dessert will be served, it's all I can think of. Then when I get it, I'm afraid I'm not getting enough; I feel fear and panic.*

- *I use eating sugar to punctuate every part of my day, in between things, when I begin or end things, etc.*

- *Even if I'm full after a meal, I feel restless and want sugar.*

- *I feel physically hung over until I can get an adequate amount of sugar first thing in the morning.*

- *Regardless of what I want to eat or think I'll eat, I eat binge foods every day.*

- *I often feel hungrier after a meal than before. Food doesn't satisfy me.*

- *I can only stop eating binge foods when they're entirely gone. If I can't manage/don't want to finish it, I'm overwhelmed with disgust at the reality of what and how much I've eaten. I try to get rid of the rest. If I leave it or throw it in the trash, I'll come back for it a bit later. Even if I dump my ashtray on it. The only thing I can do is throw it down the incinerator, which I end up regretting later when I want it again.*

- *I can't stop gaining weight. I desperately want to lose weight and can't.*

- *I can't force myself to cook for myself or eat vegetables.*

- *I can't follow a diet, even from a doctor.*

- *I can't will myself to go a day without sugar. Once I went twelve days, but I was eating 1-2 boxes of "all fruit" ice pops a day.*

- *I feel too sluggish and depressed after a binge, or eating binge food, to do anything but lie on the couch or sleep.*

- *I'll spend a significant amount of money on delivery and fees to reorder my binge food multiple times.*

- *I'll order double of what I want to ensure I don't run out before I lose interest.*

- *If I'm buying binge foods out, I need to also buy something I can eat on the way home to eat the binge food, so I'm not without the food for a moment.*

Ginger was clearly aware that she was powerless over food and that her life was unmanageable. However, she believed this intellectually but could not see herself as being powerless about this way of viewing herself.

In Dr. Vera Tarman's book, *Food Junkies*, the case study in the opening chapter discusses a man who was mostly confined to his bed and died unable to find his way into recovery.[272]

IV. The Critics

Many people in the medical and therapeutic communities still believe quite strongly that it is not a good idea to focus on the issue of powerlessness regarding food or anything else. They say, "These folks already do not think positively about themselves; focusing on being powerless only reinforces an unhealthy negative self-image."[273] This argument is often coupled with another statement, that food addiction is not a real biochemical disease. The science is now overwhelming that at least some people *do* have a substance use disorder regarding food. [274]

In response to the critics, no one sets out to have physical cravings, mental compulsions, or an addictive mind. However, food addicts *do* have these conditions to greater and lesser degrees. If one assumes that these conditions should be or can be resisted by reason and controlled by the power of will, it is eventually not going to work; and as the disease progresses, this situation will produce more and more toxic shame. On the other hand, if foods addicts can see themselves as powerless over a real biochemical disease, they can begin to heal their self-image and let go of toxic shame.

It is empowering for food addicts to realize they can ask for help and accept support from others, then accomplish goals they couldn't meet by themselves.

V. Powerful Actions for Food Addicts

- Identify and eliminate toxic foods.

In early stages of the disease, it is necessary for food addicts to identify the foods that are toxic to them. Some need to do this repetitively because the cravings keep fooling them. In early recovery, restating this repetitively to other food addicts creates a habit of mind. Spiritually, repetition is the only form of permanence; so the food addict can adopt self-disclosure as a spiritual practice. Hearing long-term food addicts doing this is especially helpful for those new to recovery, and this becomes a service recovered food addicts practice which also creates insurance for their own long-term recovery.

- Develop a habit of rigorous self-disclosure.

In the middle stages of addiction, it is not uncommon for the disease to be more advanced. Besides physical cravings, most also develop mental obsessions. At this stage, food addicts need others in recovery to be fair witness to their potentially irrational thinking. The rule of thumb is often to share with a therapist, support group, or Twelve Step sponsor thoughts you most do not want to share, and not to make decisions about food and other recovery issues. One of the more courageous actions for food addicts is to be open to help in challenging their own denial.

- Humble yourself to ask for and accept help.

In the late and final stages of food addiction, there is an even deeper level of powerlessness. Sometimes advanced food addicts cannot even imagine what it would take to put food abstinence and recovery first in their lives. They see this as being "impractical" or "unrealistic," or they see themselves as being "hopeless" or "not having the willingness" to eliminate their binge foods completely or go to any length for their own health and spiritual recovery.

Most food addicts cannot face advanced powerlessness by themselves. One of the best sources of hope is finding other food addicts who have recovered. Recovered food addicts have faced the same hopeless experiences but now have proven that there is a solution for hopelessness that is practical and realistic. Paradoxically, it is the solution, for many, of identifying and accepting powerlessness.[275]

Those of us working in the addiction model see food addiction as a biochemical disease, a medical problem just like diabetes or cancer or schizophrenia. It cannot be willed away. Most people no longer think it is shameful to have these diseases; but a few decades ago, the general population definitely did consider them shameful, and some still do. What is important in identifying powerlessness in food addiction is seeing the disease for what it is.

As mentioned above, no one sets out to have physical cravings, mental compulsions or an addictive mind. However, food addicts *do* have these conditions to greater and lesser degrees. If one assumes that these conditions should be or can be resisted by reason and controlled by the power of will, it is eventually not going to work; and as the disease progresses, this situation will produce more and more toxic shame. If food addicts say they are powerless and still feel shameful, then they are not understanding what powerlessness really is. Just like most people need help from the medical community to deal with diabetes, cancer, and schizophrenia, people also need appropriate help to deal with food addiction.

In fact, like with alcoholism and other addictions, food addicts often need extraordinary support. If the cravings have progressed, they might even need 24/7 detoxification support to go through physical withdrawal. If the mental obsessions have progressed, they often need a therapeutic or Twelve Step support group to keep taking constructive action in spite of what their addictive minds are telling them. If the addictive personality has progressed, they may need support to do deep emotional and spiritual work towards a transformation of personality. Here is the point: It is empowering to realize and difficult for food addicts to accept that they may not, probably cannot, do this alone.

An important difference between food addiction and entirely physical problems like obesity or primarily psychological problems like eating disorders is that biochemical food addictive denial is a part of food addiction. Without developing the nature of this problem completely, the important point here is that food addiction, like other chemical dependencies, is a disease that makes you forget that you have a disease. When the disease develops to this stage, the food addict is REALLY powerless to heal simply by thinking positively and working very hard. Food addicts need to find hope and work hard; but if they try to do this alone, the results are eventually likely to be not just failure, but also more and deeper toxic shame. So the usual approaches to inspiring confidence and increasing self-esteem alone do not do the job. They are counterproductive.

Thus, an important first step and continuing strategy for healing is to focus on being clear that self-reliance may work for a while, and it always has to be a PART of the recovery plan; but self-reliance alone fails us. Further, since this is part of what food addicts keep forgetting or subtly lying to themselves about and believing the lie, it is actually deeply empowering to be clear very specifically about what food addicts cannot do or change.

A major reason for the obesity epidemic is that many of the overweight and obese are also food addicted, and they need to begin by understanding that diets don't work. A reason why many eating disorders are so "treatment resistant" is that they are not JUST eating disorders; they are also misdiagnosed and mistreated food addiction, and using CBT to resolve underlying issues will not result is these people's ability to eat all foods, especially personally addictive foods, in moderation.

So we see rationale for rigorous and persistent work by food addicts to admit and accept that they are powerless over specific food(s), their thoughts about eating, and even their basic assumptions about themselves regarding food and control. There is more.

Getting the words right is important, but not sufficient. Food addicts can easily say they are powerless over sugar, for example, while still feeling guilty and ashamed for taking back their binge food over and over again. They are saying that they are powerless, but they do not really get it, so a facilitator of recovery work must pay attention to the non-verbals and the resulting action.

This is an important and long discussion which will have to wait for another time and place. However, it raises an issue that we must be conscious of when teaching about powerlessness over food and responding to initial admission of powerlessness in food addict qualifications and in the initial introductions at the beginning of ACORN (now SHiFT) workshops.[276] This is not an issue that can be or should be worked entirely with this little exercise, but it does present information as to the recovery state of food addicts and issues which are still unresolved. Occasionally the introduction time even provides an opportunity for useful feedback and opportune work on the deeper issues of food addiction denial.

THE LIMITS OF SCIENCE

Good information and arguments about the nature of food addiction are not enough if those with the disease of food addiction don't believe that it applies to them. Objective data and scientific research have proven insufficient to challenge food addiction denial. This is true for all addictions.

- Smokers who are addicted to nicotine can be shown X-rays of their lungs and provided with data about mortality rates for smokers, but this is frequently insufficient to convince an individual smoker to stop using cigarettes. Further, when they do want to stop smoking, they are frequently unable to do so.

- With all good intentions, alcoholics will often commit to stop getting drunk. The consequences of their drinking have been repeatedly very negative, they have read all the literature, their doctor has explained the likely medical consequences, and they are desperate to stop; but when they learn this means not drinking any alcohol at all for the rest of their lives, their resolve wanes.

- Before picking up drugs, most drug addicts have seen countless drug prevention information, both in writing and on TV. They have heard that addiction is progressive and that over time, they could lose all that matters to them. In spite of all this, they still pick up; and even after they started, they become convinced that they will be the exception.

Food addiction is exactly the same. Most food addicts begin gaining weight and find out they cannot take the weight off and keep it off. When they become open to the possibility that they are addicted to specific foods, they cannot imagine a life without sugar or their other "favorite" foods. In this and other books, the scientific information about food addiction is now available to many of these food addicts, but such objective challenges to food addiction denial leave them still unwilling or unable to quit.

This raises the question: What type of support do addicts, including food addicts, need to effectively challenge their own denial? In clinical terms, this is often referred to as "extraordinary support." Some choose to call this level of support "the spiritual solution." This is an essential part of food addiction treatment, and it is so subtle and complex that it requires a book of its own.

In practical terms, when the physical cravings of food addiction reach a critical level, they overpower the natural instincts of hunger and satiation. At the same time, diseased impulses in the pleasure center of the brain further distort the food addict's thinking in the cognitive center, memory center, and executive center of the brain. Over time, a cluster of these distorted thoughts combine with neurotic thinking from unresolved prior personal and social trauma. Traditional talk therapy can temporarily correct this thinking, but this seldom works in the long term if the disease has not been interrupted with complete abstinence from addictive foods and if the abstinent food addict does not have ongoing personal support from others who have a strong recovery consciousness.

It is helpful to see this as a solution which combines objective science and extraordinary support. The science includes identifying the foods that create physical craving, i.e., false starving, and eliminating them completely from the diet. It also includes identifying mental compulsions, i.e., false thinking, and surrendering to support from professionals and/or peers with stable food addiction recovery.

Frequently, active food addicts also have problems from unresolved prior trauma and/or other mental illness. The distorted physical cravings and addictive thinking become integrated with the neurotic and irrational thinking of these other illnesses. This phenomenon is frequently described as an "addictive personality." The solution is an entire "psychic change." This is sometimes referred to as a change of personality, as a spiritual experience,[277] or as reinforcing a higher recovery consciousness. As in the treatment of alcoholism and drug addiction, this is often seen as the "miracle" of recovery.

Ten Correct Statements about Addiction to Specific Food

Statement One: Food Addiction is a brain disease, and there is consensus among scientists that specific foods can be addictive.

Statement Two: The disease of food addiction can be treated successfully at each of its stages by adapting the model used for alcoholism and other drug addictions.

Statement Three: Over time, sugar and other hyper-processed foods create physical craving which can be curtailed by complete abstinence from these foods.

Statement Four: The body can obtain all the sugar it needs by eating healthy whole fruits and vegetables and by eliminating processed foods containing sugar.

Statement Five: Some people are able to lose weight and maintain it by diet and exercise, but not those with an eating disorder or food addiction.

Statement Six: Food addicts need "extraordinary support" to achieve and maintain food abstinence. This can be achieved through peer-based support, by therapist-based support, or by professional treatment.

Statement Seven: There is substantial evidence that food addiction can be treated effectively. This can be substantiated by various Twelve Step organizations and by outcome research done by various food addiction treatment programs.

Statement Eight: The progression of food addiction leads to serious physical, psychological, and spiritual illness. Untreated food addicts develop a pattern of lying not only about food, but about many other aspects of their lives.

Statement Nine: Bariatric surgery does not necessarily work for food addicts. As with alcoholism and other drug addictions, the most effective and inexpensive treatment for food addiction is Twelve Step facilitation.

Statement Ten: Becoming conscious of one's personal powerlessness over specific foods and food thoughts is essential to understanding the disease and recovering from food addiction.

BIOCHEMICAL FOOD ADDICTION DENIAL
PHYSICAL CRAVING, MENTAL OBSESSION, ADDICTED PERSONALITY

In this book's main text, I wrote about **Cognitive Food Addiction Denial**, where the facts are not true and the arguments are irrational. Another characteristic of Cognitive Food Addiction Denial is that the problems for the food addict and for the counselor are essentially conscious and rational. The solution for Cognitive Food Addiction Denial is primarily educational: identify false thinking, and replace it with what is accurate.

Biochemical Food Addiction Denial operates predominantly at the level of the unconscious. Thus, food addicts not only act on false beliefs, but also, they do not know what they don't know, *and* their misunderstandings are not very susceptible to rational correction.

The three characteristics of biochemical denial are **physical craving, mental obsession**, and **addictive personality**. Each of these is caused by an addictive food literally changing the biochemistry of the brain.

Physical craving is complicated. It develops when a potentially addictive food interacts with a predisposed part of the brain's frontal lobe. This causes a progressive chemical change in the dopamine neurotransmitters which, in turn, creates a physical dependency. At that point, *the brain starts to act like it needs more and more of the same food in order to survive.*

The physical craving experienced by the food addict <u>slowly overrides natural hunger</u>. *Natural hunger* tells the body there is a need for *nutrition.*

Craving tells the body that it <u>needs</u> the addictive food <u>immediately</u> for *survival* – even though this is not true. *Craving* can be understood as a growing experience of *false starving*. Food addicts hardly know anything has happened, but they think that they <u>*have to*</u> <u>*eat*</u>.

The food addict confuses physical craving with normal hunger. Even though there are strong negative consequences to overeating, (e.g., gaining unwanted weight and the potential for a number of serious secondary diseases), mindful reasoning is of little help in discerning this craving from healthy hunger. The most effective solution to physical craving is to completely eliminate the specific foods that are craved. Then, after a period of withdrawal (during which the food addict sometimes experiences stronger craving, as well as fatigue, anxiety, restlessness, etc.), the cravings go away.

Long before the cravings go into remission, food addicts will often strongly exert their will and try to stop gaining weight, usually because their doctor has told them weight loss will relieve high blood pressure, return a healthy balance of insulin, and prevent the onset of many other serious health problems. Because the food addict's vanity is concerned with being fat and the impression their body makes on others, their brain has to come up with a reason that it's OK to eat the trigger foods. The instinctive part of the food addict's brain engages other parts of the brain (the pleasure center, the cognitive center, the memory center, the executive center) to rationalize overeating. This is not conscious, but rather, an *unconscious* search for anything that will keep the food addict eating. These are **mental obsessions**.

Physical cravings create a situation where food addicts cannot stop eating once they start. **Mental obsessions** create a state of consciousness where the food addict cannot stop starting to overeat again. This is **addictive personality**. As both of the brain disturbances increase, the food addict is powerless – even though the ego will adamantly assert that this is impossible. This condition is doubly resistant to common sense or to talk therapy.

The reason for the craving and obsession is mainly that the person has the brain chemistry of a food addict, which is **food addiction**. The only solution that consistently works in overcoming food addiction is coming to depend on a power beyond the self.

Recovering food addicts increasingly cannot make healthy decisions about their food – or about other parts of their lives – by themselves, so they learn to consciously depend on a healthy friend to assist them in their decision-making regarding food. When that does not work, they enlist a health professional. When that does not work, they decide to take direction from a sponsor or from a group in recovery from food addiction. In doing this, they re-engage the spiritual part of themselves and, as it is put in the Twelve Step rooms, surrender to God *as they understand God.*

The solution is complex, but the central problem is simple: food addicts come to confuse the addicted part of the brain with their true selves. *In mental obsession, the food addict cannot tell if a reason for eating is true or false.* When in their addictive personality, food addicts develop a distorted notion of self. "I chose to eat out of control" rather than "the disease of food addiction hijacked my brain."

Food addiction is ultimately a spiritual problem; recovery is ultimate a transformation of personality.

In the next appendix, we will discuss *Social/Institutional Food Addiction Denial* regarding food.

SOCIAL/INSTITUTIONAL FOOD ADDICTION DENIAL

Previously, I discussed **cognitive food addiction denial**, where factual information is incorrect and reasoning is faulty, and **biochemical food addiction denial**, where specific foods themselves distort individuals' brains. There is a third important level of denial, **institutional food addiction denial**, where people with power in institutions central to our society's food supply hurt consumers (sometimes intentionally, sometimes unintentionally), and then come up with arguments to normalize these practices and build them into the woodwork such that the very fabric of society becomes toxic.

Here is one important example. When I was growing up, I, as well as most people, thought of sugar as just another _food_. As the food business changed and I became better informed, I thought of sugar more as an _additive_ or a _spice_. As time went on, we all began to learn that consumption of sugar was doing damage to our teeth, causing unwanted weight gain, and, secondarily, aggravating heart disease, certain cancers, and, most recently, COVID 19.

Yet the average adult eats four to five times as much sugar (30 teaspoons per day) as health professionals say is healthy (6-8 teaspoons per day). Despite government guidelines and parents' urging, the amount of sugar we eat continues to grow, along with the American waistline.

Approximately 80% of all processed foods in grocery stores now contain sugar (up from 20% thirty years ago), and the most recent science finds that _sugar is addictive_. Noted experts estimate that over 70 million

U.S. adults experience food cravings and loss of control related to sugar and other basic food substances. Big Food knows this and actively uses sugar, salt and fat as active ingredients in their marketing to the public. The SUBSTANCE, the DISTORTED THINKING, and the ADDICTION are baked into society. This is **Institutional Food Addiction Denial**. It is the air we breathe. Even when we know something is wrong, we don't really challenge it. It is what is real.

Business leaders, high government officials, and social critics suggested the industry cut back on the amount of sugar in their products (5% a year for each of ten years), but the answer was "No!" Institutional sugar pushers continue to sell "what people will buy," and, of course, the potentially addictive foods are heavily advertised, including to children. Almost every breakfast cereal, is *sweetened*. More problematic, this practice, and the industry's right to do it, are generally accepted. "Sweet" is more addictive than cocaine; but no one, including me, is calling for sugar to be made illegal – just *regulated*.

What are some actions we can and should take?

First, like cigarettes, densely-sugared products should have Warning Labels:"This product may be dangerous to your health."

Second, like alcoholic beverages, potentially addictive foods should be taxed with the revenue used to support public education and treatment.

Third, ultra-processed foods should be in a separate aisle in grocery stores, and minors should be prohibited from buying the most dangerously addictive food products.

We need to establish some catchy-titled grass-roots organizations (Food Addiction Upstarts) at the local and federal levels.

And we can do much more:

1. Introduce food addiction education into the school and higher-education curriculum.

2. Change the FDA's formal classification of sugar to that of a condiment, rather than that of a food.

3. Provide incentives for the food industry to minimize hyper-refining in food processing.

4. Restrict childhood use, tax adult use of addictive foods, and provide funding for food addiction treatment programs.

5. Institute special programs for military recruitment and training, correction programs, and food addiction research on food addiction treatment outcomes.

6. Revise the DSM-5 and ICD-11 guidelines to include food addiction as a disease.

LOCALLY

- **Food Addiction Councils** – or seats on local drug addiction and alcoholism councils, local research

- **Non-Addictive Cooking** – parent education hosted by churches, PTAs, hospitals, and social agencies

- **Schools and Colleges** – "Normal Eater, Emotional Eater, Food Addict," Food Addiction Prevention, Food Addiction Studies, professional training

- **Ladder of Food Addiction Treatment** – counselors, hosts for food Twelve Step meetings, inexpensive detox, recovery groups, residential treatment

- **"Food Addict Friendly"** Local Government Officials

NATIONALLY

- **Center for Disease Control (CDC)** – annual surveys of food addiction by stage and demographic group

- **American Psychiatric Association (APA)** – food addiction an official disease in DSM-5

- **Health Insurance Industry** – Reimbursement for food addiction prevention and treatment

- **Food Industry** – funding for food addiction prevention and research, 5% less sugar in all products yearly for ten years

- **Alcoholism and Drug Institute** – continued funding for basic research, treatment outcome research, and addictive properties of food additives

- **Food and Drug Administration (FDA)** – regulation of hyper-processed foods, warning labels on potentially addictive foods, none in food machines

- **Military** – include food-addiction-free eating in basic training program for overweight recruits, similar program of outreach to potential new recruits

- **Food Addiction Treatment** – hospital-based primary treatment in every state, connected to research university

- Required Abstinent Menu in Restaurants

- **Prisons** – Sugar-Free Menu and Food Addiction Recovery Pods

- Food Stamps for Abstinent Foods

- Crop Subsidies for Vegetables and Fruits

- Abstinent Food Options in Cinema, Sporting Events and Large Entertainment Complexes

- Continuing Education for Physicians, Therapists, and Dieticians

To many this would seem an overwhelming list, but so did Warning Labels on cigarettes and the idea of smoke-free businesses and public spaces just a couple of decade ago. (So did the idea of AIDS patients organizing to pressure the government and drug industry to find medicine for HIV.)

My bet is that direct action for food addiction recovery will continue to evolve as food addicts, their allies, and health professionals begin to organize locally and nationally. Until this happens, abstinent and recovered food addicts will individually have to do battle with a food-addicted society. The alternative is to challenge Institutionalized Food Addiction Denial as we also eliminate Cognitive and Biochemical Food Addiction Denial.

©copyright Phil Werdell, 2022

APPENDIX C

BIBLIOGRAPHY

I. Primary Recovery Resources

Alcoholics Anonymous, 4th ed. (2001)., *Alcoholics Anonymous: How Many Thousands of Men and Women Have Recovered from Alcoholism.* New York: Alcoholics Anonymous World Service, Inc.

Alcoholics Anonymous (2002). *Twelve Steps and Twelve Traditions.* NY: Alcoholics Anonymous World Services, Inc.

Food Addicts Anonymous, *Food Addicts Anonymous,* West Palm Beach, FL: Food Addicts Anonymous, Inc. For more information: https:// faacanhelp.org/

Food Addicts in Recovery Anonymous (2015). *Food Addicts in Recovery Anonymous.* Woburn, MA: Food Addicts in Recovery Anonymous, Inc. Available from Food Addicts in Recovery Anonymous, 400 W. Cummings Park, Suite 1700, Woburn, MA 01801, (781) 932-6300 https://www.foodaddicts.org

GreySheeters Anonymous, *12 Steps & 12 Traditions of GreySheeters Anonymous,* available from https://www.greysheet.org

Overeaters Anonymous (2018). *The Twelve Steps and Twelve Traditions of Overeaters Anonymous.* Rio Rancho, NM: Overeaters Anonymous, Inc.

Overeaters Anonymous (1980). *Overeaters Anonymous, Vol. I* Rio Rancho, NM: Overeaters Anonymous, Inc.

Overeaters Anonymous (2001). *Overeaters Anonymous, Vol. II.* Rio Rancho, NM: Overeaters Anonymous, Inc.

II. Secondary Sources on Food Addiction

Appleton, N. (1996). *Lick the Sugar Habit.* New York: Penguin Putnam.

Avena, N.M. & Talbott, J.R. (2014). *Why Diets Fail: Because You're Addicted to Sugar.* Berkeley: Ten Speed Press. Dr. Avena's research on sugar may be found on her website, drnicoleavena.com

Barnard, Neal (2003). *Breaking the Food Seduction: The Hidden Reasons behind Food Cravings—and 7 Steps to End Them Naturally.* New York: St. Martin's Press.

Brownell, K. & Gold, M. (Eds.) (2012). *Food and Addiction: A Comprehensive Manual.* New York: Oxford University Press.

Danowski, D. (2002). *Locked Up for Eating Too Much: The Diary of a Food Addict in Rehab.* Center City, MN: Hazelden.

Dufty, W. (1975). *Sugar Blues.* New York: Warner Books.

Hollis, J. (1996). *Fat is a Family Affair.* Center City, MN: Hazelden Publishing & Educational Services.

Hyman, M., *The Blood Sugar Solution: The UltraHealthy Program for Losing Weight, Preventing Disease and Feeling Great Now!* Little Brown, New York, NY, 2012

Ifland, J., Marcus, M., & Preuss, H. (2020). *Processed Food Addiction: Foundations, Assessment and Recovery,* CRC Press, New York, 2020.

Katherine, A. (1996). *Anatomy of a Food Addiction: The Brain Chemistry of Overeating,* Carlsbad, CA: Gurze Books.

Kessler, D. A. (2009). *The End of Overeating: Taking Control of the Insatiable American Appetite.* New York: Rodale.

Lerner, M. (2013). *A Guide to Eating Disorder Recovery: Defining the Problem and Finding the Solution.* Cooper City, FL: Milestones in Recovery.

McCarty, T. (2012). *Shades of Hope: How to Treat Your Addiction to Food.* New York: Berkley Books.

Nakken, C. (1996). *The Addictive Personality: Understanding the Addictive Process and Compulsive Behavior.* Center City, MN: Hazelden.

Prager, M. (2010). *Fat Boy: Thin Man.* Available on Amazon..

Pretlow, R. A. (2009). *Overweight: What Kids Say. What's Really Causing the Childhood Obesity Epidemic?* North Charleston, SC: CreateSpace.

Roth, G. (1982). *Feeding the Hungry Heart: The Experience of Compulsive Eating,* New York, New American Library.

Sheppard, K. (1993). *Food Addiction: The Body Knows.* Deerfield Beach, FL: Health Communications, Inc.

Stapleton, C. (2017). *Weight Loss Surgery Does Not Treat Food Addiction.* Mind Body Health Services Inc.

Tarman, V. with Werdell, P. (2014). *Food Junkies: The Truth about Food Addiction.* Toronto: Dundurn. Available on Amazon.

Taubes, G. (2017). *The Case Against Sugar.* New York: Knopf Doubleday Publishing Group.

Thompson, S. P. (2017). *Bright Line Eating: The Science of Living Happy, Thin, and Free.* New York: Hay House, Inc.

Twerski, A. (1997). *Addictive Thinking: Understanding Self-Deception.* Center City, MN: Hazelden.

Warren, R., et al. (2013). *The Daniel Plan: 40 Days to a Healthier Life.* Published by The Daniel Plan and available at www.zondervan.com/ebooks

Werdell, P. (2009). *Bariatric Surgery & Food Addiction: Preoperative Considerations.* Sarasota, FL: Evergreen. Available on Amazon.

Yudkin, J. (1972). *Sweet and Dangerous.* New York: Peter H Wyden.

OTHER BOOKS AND ARTICLES ON FOOD ADDICTION BY PHIL WERDELL

Werdell, P. (2021). *The Disease Concept of Food Addiction: A Story for People Interested in Recovery.* Available on Amazon.

Rocchio, B. and Werdell, P. (2017). Treating Food Addiction, The Basics—Nature, Assessment, and Principles of Treatment. Sarasota, FL: Evergreen. Available on Amazon.

Cheren, M., and Werdell, P. (2015). *A Tool Kit for Food Addiction Assessment and Treatment; the Basics from A to Z.* www.foodaddictioninstitute.org and www.umassmed.edu/psychiatry

Tarman, V. with Werdell, P. (2014). Food Junkies: The Truth about Food Addiction. Toronto: Dundurn. Available on Amazon.

Werdell, P. (2012). "From the Front Lines: Food Addiction Treatment," in Brownell and Gold (eds.), *Food and Addiction: A Comprehensive Manual.* NY: Oxford University Press

Foushi, M. and Werdell, P. (2012), *Food Plans for Food Addiction Recovery: A Physical and Spiritual Tool.* Sarasota, FL: Evergreen. Available on Amazon.

Werdell, P. (2011). Inventorying Food Slips, Physically, Mentally and Spiritually—A Practical Tool for Food Addiction Recovery. (Preface by Beth Rocchio, MD). Sarasota, Florida: Evergreen. Available on Amazon.

Werdell, P. (2009). *Bariatric Surgery & Food Addiction: Preoperative Considerations.* Sarasota, FL: Evergreen. Available on Amazon.

Cheren, M., Werdell, P., et al. (2009). *Physical Craving and Food Addiction: A Review of the Science.* Food Addiction Institute, www.foodaddictioninstitute.org

Werdell, P., Foushi, M., Weldon, C. (2007). *The ACORN Primary Intensive: A New Model of Professional Support for Food Addiction Recovery.* Sarasota, FL: Evergreen. Available on Amazon.

Werdell, P. (1994). "Beyond Traditional Eating Disorders: Food Addiction" in the *Clinical Forum* of the International Association of Eating Disorder Professionals (IAEDP).

Outcome Research on Food Addiction Treatment, with Mary DiSanzo (forthcoming)

Endnotes

Notes

1 Werdell, P. (2019). Healing Food Addiction: What Works? Outcome Evidence on Self-Help, Twelve Step Programs, and Professional Treatment, Sarasota, FL: Evergreen (forthcoming).

2 Szalavitz, M. "Can Food Really Be Addictive? Yes, Says National Drug Expert." Time Magazine, April 5, 2012. Retrieved from http://healthland.time.com/2012/04/05/yes-food-can-be-addictive-says-the-director-of-the-national-institute-on-drug-abuse/

3 One famous example was actress Gloria Swanson and her friend William Dufty who wrote Sugar Blues, Warner Books. New York, NY, 1976. Also, Werdell, op cit.

4 Other food abstinence-based Twelve Step fellowships include Food Addicts Anonymous (FAA) Compulsive Overeaters Anonymous HOW (CEA HOW), Food Addicts in Recovery Anonymous (FA). And Recovering Food Addicts Anonymous (RFA),

5 See institutional self-studies of OA 1981, 1992, 2002, 2010, 2017 and of FA 1911, 2016. Also, Werdell, op cit.

6 Hospital-based primary programs closed in 1996 when health insurance stopped reimbursing residential treatment, but we have outcome research on one of these programs:

Carroll, T. (1993). *Eating Disorder Inventory and other Predictors of Successful Symptom Management in Bulimic and Obese Women Following an Inpatient Treatment Program Employing an Addictions Paradigm,* Department of Psychological and Social Foundations, University of Florida, Tampa, FL; See also:

Hillock, Prager and Werdell, "Survey of ACORN Outcomes, 2006" in Foushi, Weldon and Werdell. (2007). *Food Addiction Recovery, A New Model of Professional Support – The ACORN Primary Intensive,* Evergreen Publications (Amazon), Sarasota, FL; and

Olofdotter, O. (2017). "Survey of (Out-Patient Food Addiction Program) MFM Outcomes" in manuscript form (2019), MFM, Reykjavik, Iceland. See also,

Werdell, op cit. Note: Other food Addiction treatment programs include Milestone of Miami, Turning Point of Tampa, Renaissance of Toronto, Shades of Hope of Texas, Raja's Center in Jordon, and PROMIS in Great Britain.

7 Ifland, et al, "Refined Food Addiction: A Classic Substance Use Disorder." Medical Hypothesis, 72, 518-526, 2009; Sheppard, K. (1993). Food Addiction: The Body Knows. Deerfield Beach, FL: Health Communications;

Danowski, D. (2009) *Why Can't I Stop Eating So Much?* Minneapolis, MN: Hazelden.

8 Avena, N., et al. (2008). "Evidence of Sugar Addiction: Behavioral and Neurochemical Effects of intermittent, Excessive Sugar Intake" Neuroscience and Biobehavioral Reviews, pp 20-39.

9 CASA (2016), "Understanding and Addressing Food Addiction: A Scientific Approach to Policy, Practice and Research," published by the National Center on Addiction and Substance Abuse (CASA). This paper is available at https://www.centeronaddiction.org/addiction-research/reports/understanding-and-addressing-food-addiction-science-based-approach-policy

10 Gold, M. (ed.) (2004). Eating Disorders, Overeating and Pathological Attachment to Food: Independent of Addictive Disorders? New York, NY: Hathaway.

11 www.usgov/nida.

12 Noble, E., et al., "D2 Dopamine Receptor Gene and Obesity," International Journal of Eating Disorders, Vol 15, No 3, April, 1994.

13 Cheren, M., et al. (2009). "Physical Craving and Food Addiction: A Review of the Science," Food Addiction Institute, www.foodaddictioninstitue.org. This paper suggests there may be Type I food addicts and Type II food addicts. Type I are genetically predis-

posed; Type II become addicted primarily through environmental causes.

14 Drewnowski, A., et al. (1992). "Taste response and Preferences for Sweet High-Fat Foods: Evidence of Opioid Involvement." Physical Behavior, 51: p 71-9.

15 These medications have been tested, offering some help for Binge Eating Disorder, but have not been tested for food addiction:

Vyvanse lisdexamfetamine dimesylate, fluoxetine. Source: https://www.drugs.com/mtm/lisdexamfetamine.html

Topiramate (Topamax). Source: https://www.webmd.com/drugs/2/drug-14494-6019/topamax-oral/topiramate-oral/details/list-conditions

16 Gearhardt, A., et al. "Preliminary Validation of the Yale Food Addiction Scale, Appetite, 53(2). 430-536, 2009. Not all eating disorders have a food addiction component.

17 Colantuoni, C., et al. (2002). "Evidence That Intermittent Excessive Sugar Intake Causes Endogenous Opioid Dependence," Obesity Research.

18 Lustig, R. (2013). Fat Chance: Beating the Odds Against Sugar, Processed Food, Obesity and Disease. New York: Hudson St Press.

19 Ahmed, S., "Is Sugar as Addictive as Cocaine? in Food Addiction: The Obesity Epidemic Connection, Islandwood, Bainbridge Island, WA or www.obesityfoodaddicctionsymposium.com.

20 Moss, M. (2013). Salt, Sugar, Fat: How the Food Giants Hooked Us, New York: Random House

21 Kessler, D. (2009). The End of Overeating: Taking Control of the Insatiable American Appetite, New York: Rodale.

22 See Werdell, P. (2019). Healing Food Addiction: What Works? Outcome Evidence on Self-Help, Twelve Step Programs, and Professional Treatment, Sarasota, FL: Evergreen.

23 Brian Hoffmann (Medical College of Wisconsin, Medical College of Wisconsin, Medical College of Wisconsin, Marquette University), George Ronan (Medical College of Wisconsin, Marquette University), Dhanush Haspula (Medical College of Wisconsin), "The Influence of Sugar and Artificial Sweeteners on Vascular Health during the Onset and Progression of Diabetes." Study presented at the 2018 Experimental Biology meeting, 2018. Board # / Pub #: A322 603.20

Smith, D. G., & Robbins, T. W. (2013). The neurobiological underpinnings of obesity and binge eating: A rationale for adopting the food addiction model. Biological Psychiatry, 73(9), 804-810.

Davis, C., Loxton, N. J., Levitan, R. D., Kaplan, A. S., Carter, J. C., & Kennedy, J. L. (2013). 'Food addiction' and its association with a dopaminergic multilocus genetic profile. Physiology and Behavior.

Doi:10.1016/.physbeh.2013.05.014.

211 Davis, C., Levitan, R. D., Kaplan, A. S., Kennedy, J. L., & Carter, J. C. (2014). Food cravings, appetite, and snack-food consumption in response to a psychomotor stimulant drug: The moderating effect of "food-addiction". Frontiers in Psychology, 5(Article 403). doi:10.3389/fpsyg.2014.00403.

212 Smith, D. G., & Robbins, T. W. (2013). The neurobiological underpinnings of obesity and binge eating: A rationale for adopting the food addiction model. Biological Psychiatry, 73(9), 804-810. Wise, R. A. (2013). Dual roles of dopamine in food and drug seeking: The drive-reward paradox. Biological Psychiatry, 73(9), 819-826.

Filbey, F. M., Myers, U. S., & DeWitt, S. (2012). Reward circuit function in high BMI individuals with compulsive overeating: Similarities with addiction. NeuroImage, 63(4), 1800-1806.

Wang, G. J., Geliebter, A., Volkow, N. D., Telang, F. W., Logan, J., Jayne, M. C., ... Fowler, J. S. (2011). Enhanced striatal dopamine release during food stimulation in binge eating disorder. Obesity

(Silver Spring), 19(8), 16011608.

Smith, D. G., & Robbins, T. W. (2013). The neurobiological underpinnings of obesity and binge eating: A rationale for adopting the food addiction model. Biological Psychiatry, 73(9), 804-810.

24 https://www.asam.org/resources/definition-of-addiction

25 www.apa.org. American Psychiatric Association Diagnostic and Statistical Manual of Mental Disorders, 5th edition.

26 Richter, L. (2016). Understanding and Addressing Food Addiction: A Scientific Approach to Policy, Practice and Research," National Center of Addiction and Substance Abuse, New Haven CT.

27 Brownell and Gold, eds. (2012). Food and Addiction: A Comprehensive Handbook. New York: Oxford University Press.

28 See the Food Addiction Institute's international educational campaign "Food addiction is real! There is a solution!" at foodaddictioninstitute.org.

29 Werdell, et al. "Physical Cravings and Food Addiction: A Review of the Science," www.foodaddictioninstitute.org. This paper was presented to the American Psychiatric Association Committees on Eating Disorders and on Substance Abuse for the DSM-5.

30 Brownell and Gold (eds.) (2012). Food and Addiction: A Comprehensive Handbook, New York: Oxford University Press.

31 Ahmed, S., "Intense Sweetness Surpasses Cocaine Reward," in Food Addiction: The Obesity Epidemic Connection, IslandWood. Bainbridge Island, WA. The sweet substance tested was artificial sweetener.

32 Hillock, Prager and Werdell, "Survey of ACORN Outcomes" in Foushi, Weldon and Werdell. (2006). Food Addiction Recovery, A New Professional Model of Professional Support, - The ACORN Primary Intensive ™, Sarasota, FL: Evergreen.

33 Dufty, W. (1975). Sugar Blues. New York: Warner Books

34 Wunderlich, R. (1982). Sugar and Your Health, St. Petersburg, FL: Good Health Publications.

35 Hollis, J. (1985). Fat Is a Family Affair. Center City, MN: Hazelden.

36 Appleton, N. (1996). Lick the Sugar Habit. New York: Avery.

37 Sheppard, K. (1989)., Food Addiction: The Body Knows, Health Communication, Deerfield Beach, FL, 1989.

38 Katherine, A. (1996). Anatomy of a Food Addiction: The Brain Chemistry of Overeating. Carlsbad, CA: Gurze Books.

39 Ifland, J. (2003). Sugars and Flours: How They Make Us Crazy, Sick and Fat and What to Do about It. 1st Books Library, www.1stbooks.com.

40 DesMaisons, K. (2000). The Sugar Addict's Total Recovery Program. New York: Random House.

41 Werdell, P. (2019). "Food Addiction Denial No. 1." A blog originally published on food addiction.com.

42 Danowski, D, and Lazaro, P. (2009). Why Can't I Stop Eating? Recognizing, Understanding, and Overcoming Food Addiction. Center City, MN: Hazelden Publishing.

43 Bernard, N. (2003). Breaking the Food Seduction: The Hidden Reasons Behind Food Cravings – and 7 Steps to End them Naturally. New York: St. Martin's Press.

44 Hyman, M. (2012). The Blood Sugar Solution: The UltraHealthy Program for Losing Weight, Preventing Disease and Feeling Great Now! New York: Little Brown.

45 Peeke, P. (2013). The Hunger Fix: The Three-Stage Detox and Recovery Plan for Overeaters and Food Addiction. NY: Rodale.

46 Tarman, V. (2018). Food Junkies: The Truth About Food Addiction, Edition No 2. Toronto: Dundurn.

47 www.oa.org

48 www.foodaddicts.org

49 www.greysheet.org

50 www.ceahow.org

51 See more detailed discussion in Denial Statement #3.

52 Werdell, P. (2012). Food Plans for Food Addiction Recovery: A Physical and Spiritual Tool, Evergreen, Sarasota, FL. The Glenbeigh Food Plan was originally called the ACORN Food Plan, standing for Addictive Concept of Overeating Recovery Needs. When the hospital program closed, ACORN Food Dependency Recovery Service suggested this food plan as a place to start for those not abstinent; but for those food addicts who had been successful using another plan in the past, they could begin with this plan. This worked for a majority of clients, partly because treatment includes support regarding the principle of spiritual surrender. See Werdell, P. (forthcoming 2022). Outcomes Research for Food Addiction Treatment, Evergreen, Sarasota, FL.

53 These food plans tend to follow a common pattern: no sugar, no flour, no alcohol, weigh and measure. OA suggests eliminating all binge foods. FAA recommends avoiding a hundred names for sugar. GreySheet eliminates most starches. RFA eliminates wheat. Weighing and measuring at each meal deals with problems of volume, and it is also a part of the spiritual surrender process.

54 Food Addicts Anonymous,"100 Names for Sugar."

55 Cheren, M, et al. (2015). "A Tool Kit for Food Addiction Assessment and Treatment for Physicians, Dietitians, Therapists and Other Allied Health Professionals," Second National Conference on Treatment of Food Addiction sponsored by the University of Massachusetts School of Medicine and the Food Addiction Institute.

56 Katherine, A. (1996). Anatomy of a Food Addiction: The Brain Chemistry of Overeating, Gurze Books, Carlsbad, CA.

57 Steward, H. Leighton, et al. (2003). The New Sugar Busters! Cutting Sugar to Trim Fat. New York: Random House.

58 Sheppard, K. (1989). Food Addiction: The Body Knows, Deerfield Beach, FL., Health Communication.

59 Deneen, Gold, and Liu. "Food Addiction and Cues in Prader-Willi," Addictive Medicine, Volume 3, Number I, 2009.

60 The obvious substances needing research are the artificial sweeteners. It would also be a good idea to research the substances on the "99 names of sugar" list in the book Food Addiction Anonymous, published by FoodAddictsAnonymous.org. A comparable list by a registered dietician is by Theresa Wright, MS, RD, LDN. (2006). "Names of Sugar." Renaissance Nutrition Center, Inc.

61 Noble, E., et al, "D2 Dopamine Receptor Gene and Obesity," International Journal of Eating Disorders, Vol. 15, No. 3, 1994.

62 An unpublished study done by the graduate students of endocrinology professor at University of California at San Francisco Robert Lustig.

63 Werdell, P., "Food Addiction Treatment: An Important Missing Piece in the Obesity Epidemic Puzzle," a keynote address at the First National Food Addiction Treatment Conference at The University of Massachusetts School of Medicine cosponsored by the Food addiction Institute, October 2014.

64 Rocchio, B., and Werdell, P. (2017). Treating Food Addiction, Book 1: The Basics—Nature, Assessment and Principles of Treatment. Sarasota FL: Evergreen.

65 American Society of Addictive Medicine, https://www.asam.org/quality-care/definition-of-addiction

66 Cheren, M., et al. (2009). "Physical Craving and Food Addiction: A Review of the Science," Food Addiction Institute, www.foodaddictioninstitue.org.

67 Tarman, V. (2018). Food Junkies: The Truth About Food Addiction, 2cond Edition, Dundurn, Toronto, CAN.

68 Silkworth, W. (2001). in "The Doctor's Opinion". Alcoholics

Anonymous: The Story of How Many Thousands of Men and Women Have Recovered from Alcoholism, Alcoholics, Fourth Edition.

69 This "volume addiction" may be due to the amount of combined sugar in the total amount of food eaten. It can also be caused by the lack of leptin, a chemical at the cellular level which controls the satiation response.

70 Brownell, K and Gold, M. (2012). Part VII "Concluding Comments" in Food and Addiction: A Comprehensive Handbook," Oxford University Press, New York, NY.

71 Silkworth, W. (1939). "The Doctor's Opinion," Alcoholics Anonymous, How Many Thousands of Men and Woman Have Recovered from Alcoholism, New York, New York: Alcoholics Anonymous Worlds Service, Inc.

72 Sheppard, K, (1989). Food Addiction: The Body Knows, Health Communications, Deerfield Beach, FL.

73 Denial Statement #2.

74 Wang, Gene-Jack, in Mark Gold (Ed.) (2004). Eating Disorders, Overeating, and Pathological Attachment to Food: Independent or Addictive Disorders? New York, Hathaway; co-published simultaneously as Journal of Addictive Diseases, Volume 23, Number 3, 2004.

75 https://www.asam.org/quality-care/definition-of-addiction.

76 The classic description of the addictive mind can be found in the chapter "More About Alcoholism" in Alcoholics Anonymous, How Many Thousands of Men and Woman Have Recovered from Alcoholism, Alcoholics Anonymous Worlds Service, Inc. New York, New York, 1939.

77 Twerski, A. (1997). Addictive Thinking: Understanding Self-Deception. Center City, MN: Hazelden.

78 Ajlouni, S. (2018). "A New Beginning: Workbook for Jordan

Food Addiction Intensive" Sachir Ajlouni, Amman, JOR.

79 Beck, J. (2008). The Beck Diet Solution: Train Your Brain to Think Like a Thin Person. Birmingham, AL: Oxmoor House.

80 Rocchio, B. and Werdell, P. (2017). Treating Food Addiction, The Basics—Nature, Assessment, and Principles of Treatment. Sarasota, FL: Evergreen. Available on Amazon.

81 Twerski, A. (1997). Addictive Thinking: Understanding Self-Deception. Center City, MN: Hazelden. See also:

Starks, C. "A Professional's Perspective" in Food Addicts Anonymous, *Food Addicts Anonymous,* West Palm Beach, FL: Food Addicts Anonymous, Inc. For more information: info@foodaddictsanonymous.org

82 These examples come from my clinical experience working with middle- and late-stage food addicts.

83 C, L. [Lawrie]. (2014). OA Big Book Study Guide for Compulsive Overeaters. lawrie@oabigbook.info.

84 C, L. [Lawrie]. (2014). OA Big Book Study Guide for Compulsive Overeaters. lawrie@oabigbook.info.

85 Twerski, A. (1997). Addictive Thinking: Understanding Self-Deception, Center City, MN: Hazelden, pp. 7-8, 34.

86 Twerski, p. 34.

87 Twerski, A. (1997). Addictive Thinking: Understanding Self-Deception, Center City, MN: Hazelden, pp. 5-7.

88 Nakken, C. (1996). The Addictive Personality: Understanding the Addictive Process and Compulsive Behavior. Center City, MN: Hazelden.

89 Alcoholics Anonymous. (2001). Alcoholics Anonymous. New York: Alcoholics Anonymous World Service, Inc., Fourth Edition.

90 Twerski, A. (1997). Addictive Thinking: Understanding Self-Deception, Center City, MN: Hazelden

91 Peeke, P. (2013). The Hunger Fix: The Three-Stage Detox and Recovery Plan for Overeaters and Food Addiction. NY: Rodale.

92 Twerski, A. (1997). Addictive Thinking: Understanding Self-Deception, Center City, MN: Hazelden.

93 Werdell, Philip, from counseling work with individual clients.

94 Werdell, Philip, from counseling work with individual clients.

95 https://www.who.int/nutrition/publications/guidelines/sugars_intake/en/ A recent nutritional advisory of the US Department of Agriculture recommended 8-12 teaspoons per day.

96 https://www.angelesinstitute.edu/thenightingale/daily-sugar-intake

97 There is no current research on the amount of sugar eaten by food addicts, but it is common sense. The most common addictive substance is sugar. Food addicts, by definition, are overeaters. Clinical observations find the consumption of food by many late-stage bulimics and binge-eating food addicts is often in excess of 3,000 calories and more.

98 Taubes, G. (2017). The Case Against Sugar. New York: Alfred A. Knopf.

99 Barnard, N. (2003). Breaking the Food Seduction: The Hidden Reasons behind Food Cravings—and 7 Steps to End Them Naturally. New York: St. Martin's Press.

100 Tarman, V., and Werdell, P. (2014). Food Junkies: The Truth about Food Addiction. Toronto: Dundurn.

101 Avena, N. and Talbott, J. (2014). Why Diets Fail: Because You're Addicted to Sugar. Berkeley: Ten Speed Press. Note: Many members of Overeaters Anonymous see themselves as "compulsive overeaters" but not as "food addicts." These individuals might have an eating disorder without a food addiction, and they might be food addicts in denial, especially if they are not stably abstinent. In these cases, there is a much wider variation in food plans. Some

food plans even include sugar and alcohol. Examples of these can be seen in the publication: Overeaters Anonymous World Service, "Dignity of Choice," Overeaters Anonymous, Inc, Rio Rancho, New Mexico, or www.oa.org

102 Heller, R. and Heller, R.F. (1991). The Carbohydrate Addict's Diet: The Lifelong Solution to Yo-Yo Dieting. New York: Dutton, Division of Penguin Books.

103 Food Addicts in Recovery Anonymous. (2015). Food Addicts in Recovery Anonymous. Woburn, MA: Food Addicts in Recovery Anonymous, Inc.; www.foodaddicts.org

104 Overeaters Anonymous—HOW, https://www.oahowphone-meetings.com/

105 Food Addicts Anonymous, "99 Names for Sugar," www.foodaddictsanonymous.org; see also: Theresa Wright, MS, RD, LDN, "Sugar," Renaissance Nutrition Center, https://sanefood.com/

106 Wright, T. in Tarman, V. and Werdell, P. (2014) Food Junkies: The Truth about Food Addiction. Toronto: Dundurn.

107 www.greysheet.org

108 Leibowitz, "Over Consumption of Fats: A Vicious Cycle from the Start." Presented at the Summit on Food Addiction: The Obesity Epidemic Connection, IslandWood, Bainbridge Island, WA, 2009.

109 Sheppard, K. (1993). Food Addiction: The Body Knows, Deerfield Beach, Florida: Health Communications, Inc.; Also: Barnard, N. (2003). Breaking the Food Seduction. New York: St. Martin's Press. See also:

  Wright, T. (2004). *Your Personal food Plan: A Basic Food Plan for Recovery from Addictive and Compulsive Eating Behaviors.* Plymouth Meeting, PA: Renaissance Nutrition Center, Inc.

110 Werdell, P. and Foushi, M. (2012). Food Plans for Food Addiction Recovery: A Physical and Spiritual Tool. Sarasota, FL: Ever-Green.

111 American Dental Association, https://www.ada.org/en

112 Appleton, N. (1996). Licking the Sugar Habit, New York: Penguin.

113 Appleton, N. and Jacobs, G.N. (2009). Suicide by Sugar: A Startling Look at Our #1 National Addiction. Garden City Park, NY: SquareOne Publishers.

114 Food Addicts Anonymous, "99 Names for Sugar," www.foodaddictsanonymous.org

115 Moss, M. (2013). Sugar, Salt, Fat: How the Food Giants Hooked Us. New York: Random House.

116 Lustig, R. (2014). Fat Chance: Beating the Odds against Sugar, Processed Food, Obesity, and Disease. New York: Penguin Group.

117 Moss, M. (2013). Sugar, Salt, Fat: How the Food Giants Hooked Us. New York: Random House.

118 CASA. (2016). "Understanding and Addressing Food Addiction: A Scientific Approach to Policy, Practice and Research," published by the National Center on Addiction and Substance Abuse (CASA).

119 Taubes, G. (2017). The Case Against Sugar. New York: Knopf Doubleday Publishing Group.

120 Ibid.

121 According to the CDC, almost 1/3 of US adults do not present with a problem of weight at all.

122 Some people are overweight primarily because of medical issues such as underactive thyroid or dysfunctional metabolism.

123 Some in early stages of food addiction are able to diet successfully for a while, but are unable to maintain the weight loss.

124 https://sciencebasedmedicine.org/calories-in-calories-out/

125 World Health Organization, 2015, as cited in Taubes, G.

(2017). The Case Against Sugar. New York: Alfred A. Knopf. Fifty years ago, one in eight American adults was obese; today the number is greater than one in three. The World Health Organization reports that obesity rates have doubled worldwide since 1980; in 2014, more than half a billion adults on the planet were obese, and more than forty million children under the age of five were overweight or obese.

126 https://www.cdc.gov/obesity/adult/defining.html

127 https://www.cdc.gov/nchs/data/factsheets/factsheet_nhanes.htm

128 Consumer Reports, "Losing Weight Your Way: 9,000 Readers Rate 13 Diet Plans and Tools," February, 2013.

129 By some estimates, 80% of people who successfully lose at least 10% of their body weight will gradually regain it to end up as large or even larger than they were before they went on a diet. Source: https://www.webmd.com › diet › how-your-appetite-can-sabotage-weight-loss

130 Fed Up the movie; Brownell, K. & Gold, M. (Eds.) (2012). Food and Addiction: A Comprehensive Manual. New York: Oxford University Press.

131 Fairburn, C. and Brownell, K. (Eds.) (2002). Eating Disorders and Obesity: A Comprehensive Handbook. New York: Guilford Press.

132 Hudson, J., Hiripi, E., Pope, H., and Kessler, R. "The Prevalence and Correlates of Eating Disorders in the National Comorbidity Survey Republican." Biological Psychiatry. Author manuscript. Available in PMC 2008 Feb 1. Published in final edited form as: Biol Psychiatry 2007 Feb 1; 61(3): 348-358. Published online 2008, Jul 3. Doi: 10.1016/j.biopsych 2006.03.040. For men, the figures are .3% anorexic, .5% bulimic, and 2.0% binge eating disorder.

Lifetime prevalence estimates of DSM-IV anorexia nervosa, bulimia nervosa, and binge eating disorder are 9%, 1.5%, and 3.5% among women, and 3%, 5%, and 2.0% among men. Survival analysis based on retrospective age-of-onset reports suggests that risk of bulimia nervosa and binge eating disorder increased with successive birth cohorts. All 3disorders are significantly comorbid with many other DSM-IV disorders. Lifetime anorexia nervosa is significantly associated with low current weight (body-mass index 18.5), whereas lifetime binge eating disorder is associated with current severe obesity (body-mass index < _ 40). Although most respondents with 12-month bulimia nervosa and binge eating disorder report some role impairment (data unavailable for anorexia nervosa since no respondents met criteria for 12-month prevalence), only a minority of cases ever sought treatment.

133 Fairburn, C. and Brownell, K. (Eds.) (2002). Eating Disorders and Obesity: A Comprehensive Handbook. New York: Guilford Press.

134 Tarman, V. and Werdell, P. (2014). Food Junkies: The Truth about Food Addiction. Toronto: Dundurn.

135 Flint, A. J., Gearhardt, A. N., Corbin, W. R., Brownell, K. D., Field, A. E., & Rimm, E. B. (2014). Food-addiction scale measurement in 2 cohorts of middle-aged and older women. American Journal of Clinical Nutrition, 99(3), 578-586.

Gearhardt, A. N., Corbin, W. R., & Brownell, K. D. (2009). Preliminary validation of the Yale Food Addiction Scale. *Appetite, 52*(2), 430-436.

Gearhardt, A. N., Boswell, R. G., & White, M. A. (2014). The association of "food addiction" with disordered eating and body mass index. *Eating Behaviors, 15*(3), 427-433.

Meule, A. (2011). How prevalent is "food addiction"? *Frontiers in Psychiatry, 2*(61), 1-4.

Meule, A., & Gearhardt, A. N. (2014). Food addiction in the light of DSM-5. *Nutrients, 6*(9), 3653-3671.

Pedram, P., Wadden, D., Amini, P., Gulliver, W., Randell, E., Cahill, F., … Sun, G. (2013). Food addiction: Its prevalence and significant association with obesity in the general population. *PLoS One, 8*(9), e74832.

Pursey, K. M., Collins, C. E., Stanwell, P., & Burrows, T. L. (2015). The stability of 'food addiction' as assessed by the Yale Food Addiction Scale in a non-clinical population over 18-months. *Appetite, 96*, 533-538. (As quoted in "Understanding and Addressing Food Addiction: A Science-Based Approach to Policy, Practice and Research, published by The National Center on Addiction and Substance Abuse [CASA], February, 2016.) Also, American' Psychiatric Association, *Diagnostic and Statistical Manual of Mental Disorders, DSM-5*, Washington, DC: American Psychiatric Publishing, 2013.

136 Pursey, K. M., Stanwell, P., Gearhardt, A. N., Collins, C. E., & Burrows, T. L. (2014). The prevalence of food addiction as assessed by the Yale Food Addiction Scale: A systematic review. Nutrients, 6(10), 4552-4590. (Also quoted in CASA; see footnote 6.)

137 Kessler, D. (2009). The End of Overeating: Taking Control of the Insatiable American Appetite. New York: Rodale Press, 2009, and

Kessler, D. (2013). *Your Food Is Fooling You: How Your Brain Is Hijacked by Sugar, Fat, and Salt.* New York: Roaring Brook Press.

138 The difference between comfort foods and trigger foods is subtle, and many who are both eating disordered and food addicted use food both ways.

139 "Understanding and Addressing Food Addiction: A Science-Based Approach to Policy, Practice and Research, published by The National Center on Addiction and Substance Abuse (CASA), February, 2016.)

140 Kessler, D. (2013). Your Food Is Fooling You: How Your Brain Is Hijacked by Sugar, Fat, and Salt. New York: Roaring Brook Press.

141 Kessler, D. (2009). The end of Overeating: Taking Control of the Insatiable American Appetite. New York: Rodale.

142 Gearhardt, A. N., White, M. A., Masheb, R. M., & Grilo, C. M. (2013). An examination of food addiction in a racially diverse sample of obese patients with binge eating disorder in primary care set-

tings. Comprehensive Psychiatry, 54(5), 500-505. Meule, A., Heckel, D., & Kubler, A. (2012). Factor structure and item analysis of the Yale Food Addiction Scale in obese candidates for bariatric surgery. European Eating Disorders Review, 20(5), 419-422. Gearhardt, A. N., Corbin, W. R., & Brownell, K. D. (2009). Preliminary validation of the Yale Food Addiction Scale. Appetite, 52(2), 430-436.

143 "Understanding and Addressing Food Addiction: A Science-Based Approach to Policy, Practice and Research, published by The National Center on Addiction and Substance Abuse [CASA], February, 2016.). Flint, A. J., Gearhardt, A. N., Corbin, W. R., Brownell, K. D., Field, A. E., & Rimm, E. B. (2014). Food-addiction scale measurement in 2 cohorts of middle-aged and older women. American Journal of Clinical Nutrition, 99(3), 578-586. Gearhardt, A. N., Boswell, R. G., & White, M. A. (2014). The association of "food addiction" with disordered eating and body mass index. Eating Behaviors, 15(3), 427-433. Meule, A. (2011). How prevalent is "food addiction"? Frontiers in Psychiatry, 2(61), 1-4. Meule, A., & Gearhardt, A. N. (2014). Food addiction in the light of DSM-5. Nutrients, 6(9), 3653-3671. Pedram, P., Wadden, D., Amini, P., Gulliver, W., Randell, E., Cahill, F., ... Sun, G. (2013). Food addiction: Its prevalence and significant association with obesity in the general population. PLoS One, 8(9), e74832. Pursey, K. M., Stanwell, P., Gearhardt, A. N., Collins, C. E., & Burrows, T. L. (2014). The prevalence of food addiction as assessed by the Yale Food Addiction Scale: A systematic review. Nutrients, 6(10), 4552-4590.

144 Center for Disease Control (CDC) https://www.cdc.gov/

145 Werdell, P. "Food Addiction Treatment: An Important Missing Piece in the Obesity Epidemic Puzzle." Keynote address at First Annual National Conference on Food Addiction, University of Massachusetts School of Medicine, October 22, 2014. A very small percentage have other medical problems, such as a thyroid deficiency.

146 Tarman, V. and Werdell, P. (2014). Food Junkies: The Truth about Food Addiction. Toronto: Dundurn.

147 Mackenzie, N. G. "Q: Why can't I ever turn down sweets? A: Blame your brain." Weight Watchers Magazine, January/February 2013, p. 40.

148 Forbes, L. (2013). "Food Addiction: An Overlooked Cause of Persistent Overweight and Obesity." Doctoral dissertation presented to the Faculty of Saybrook University, San Francisco, CA, May 2013.

149 Prose, F. (2013). Gluttony. New York: Oxford University Press, 2013.

150 Rader, W. (1980). "A Disease of the Mind"; Lindner, Peter MD, "A Disease of the Body"; Boas, R., "A Disease of the Spirit; all published in Overeaters Anonymous, Torrance, CA: Overeaters Anonymous, Inc. Also,

Starks, C. "A Professional's Perspective" in Food Addicts Anonymous, *Food Addicts Anonymous,* West Palm Beach, FL: Food Addicts Anonymous, Inc. For more information: info@foodaddictsanonymous.org

151 Consumer Reports, "Losing Weight Your Way: 9,000 Readers Rate 13 Diet Plans and Tools," February, 2013.

152 Werdell, P. (2009). Bariatric Surgery & Food Addiction: Preoperative Considerations. Sarasota, FL: EverGreen Publications. Also available on Amazon.

153 Werdell, P. "Food Addiction Treatment: An Important Missing Piece in the Obesity Epidemic Puzzle." Keynote address, First National Conference on Food Addiction Treatment, University of Massachusetts Medical School, October 22, 2014.

154 American Psychiatric Association. (2013). Diagnostic and Statistical Manual of Mental Disorders Fifth Edition (DSM-5). Washington, DC: American Psychiatric Publishing, p. 329.

155 Hudson, J.I., Hiripi, E., Pope, H.G., & Kessler, R.C, (2007). The prevalence and correlates of eating disorders in the National Comorbidity Survey Replication. Biological Psychiatry, 61(3), 348-358.

156 Roth, G. (1982). Feeding the Hungry Heart: The Experience of Compulsive Eating, New York, New American Library.

Fairburn, C. and Brownell, K. (Eds.) (2002). Eating Disorders and Obesity: A Comprehensive Handbook. New York: Guilford Press.

Fairburn and Wilson (Eds.) (1993). *Binge Eating: Nature, Assessment and Treatment.* New York: Guilford Press.

157 American Psychiatric Association. (2013). Diagnostic and Statistical Manual of Mental Disorders Fifth Edition (DSM-5). Washington, DC: American Psychiatric Publishing, p. 329. Several studies by Gearhardt found that about half of those with Binge Eating Disorder also are also positive for food addiction using the YALE Food Addiction Scale.

Gearhardt, A. N., White, M. A., & Potenza, M. N. (2011). Binge eating disorder and food addiction. Current Drug Abuse Reviews, 4(3), 201-207.

Gearhardt, A. N., White, M. A., Masheb, R. M., & Grilo, C. M. (2013). An examination of food addiction in a racially diverse sample of obese patients with binge eating disorder in primary care settings. Comprehensive Psychiatry, 54(5), 500-505.

Gearhardt, A. N., White, M. A., Masheb, R. M., Morgan, P. T., Crosby, R. D., & Grilo, C. M. (2012). An examination of the food addiction construct in obese patients with binge eating disorder. International Journal of Eating Disorders, 45(5), 657-663.

158 Shivaram, M. (2011). "Food Addiction: Assessing Withdrawal and Tolerance." Unpublished graduate dissertation supervised by Brownell, Gearhardt, and Roberto, Yale University, April 18 2011.

Kline, M. (1983). *The Junk Food Withdrawal Manual.* Denver, CO: Nutri-Books Corp.

Wideman, C.H., G.R. Nadzam, and H.M. Murphy, Implications of an animal model of sugar addiction withdrawal and relapse for human health. *Nutr Neurosci*, 2005. 8(5-6): p. 269-76.

159 Rocchio, B. and Werdell, P. (2017). Treating Food Addiction, The Basics—Nature, Assessment, and Principles of Treatment. Sarasota, FL: Evergreen. Available on Amazon.

160 Werdell, P. (2019). "Chapter 5: Qualitative Research –Incidences of Powerlessness." In Outcome Research on the Treatment of Food Addiction, Sarasota, FL: EverGreen.

161 Werdell, P. "Food Addiction Treatment: An Important Missing Piece in the Obesity Epidemic Puzzle." Keynote address, First National Conference on Food Addiction Treatment, University of Massachusetts Medical School, October 22, 2014.

162 Three residential treatment programs for eating disorders and food addiction which we recommend are: Turning Point of Tampa, Milestones in Miami, and Shades of Hope in Texas.

www.foodaddiction.com. This analysis is based on 25 years of clinical experience in SHiFT Recovery by ACORN (previously ACORN Food Dependency Recovery Services). An earlier version of this material was written for www.foodaddiction.com.

163 www.oa.com, www.overeatersanonymous.org, www.foodaddictsanonymous.org, www.foodaddicts.org, www.oahow.org, www.ceahow.org, www.recoveryfromfoodaddiction.org

164 Werdell, P. (2009). Bariatric Surgery & Food Addiction: Preoperative Considerations. Sarasota, FL: EverGreen Publications. Also available on Amazon.

165 Gearhardt, A., et al., "Preliminary validation of the Yale Food Addiction Scale, Appetite, 53(2). 430-536, 2009. Not all eating disorders have a food addiction component.

166 https://www.bittensaddiction.com/en/addiction/sugar-addiction/

167 https://www.bittensaddiction.com/en/professional-training/sugar/

168 The clinical diagnosis of Bulimia Nervosa may be found in the

APA DSM-5 (See next footnote).

169 American Psychiatric Association, Diagnostic and Statistical Manual of Mental Disorders Fifth Edition (DSM-5). Washington, DC: American Psychiatric Publishing, 2013

170 See the text of the ABA fellowship, Anorexics and Bulimics Anonymous, at www.anorexicsandbulimisanonymousaba.com.

171 Anorexics and Bulimics Anonymous, Anorexics and Bulimics Anonymous: The fellowship details its program of recovery for anorexia and bulimia. Edmonton, Albert, Canada: Anorexics and Bulimics Anonymous, 2002. ABA makes no comment on whether or not its members might be addicted to specific foods.

172 www.foodaddiction.com. This analysis is based on 25 years of clinical experience in SHiFT Recovery by ACORN (previously ACORN Food Dependency Recovery Services). An earlier version of this material was written for www.foodaddiction.com.

173 Sheppard, K. (1989). Food Addiction: The Body Knows. Deerfield Beach, FL: Health Communications, Inc.

Overeaters Anonymous. (2018). *Twelve Steps and Twelve Traditions of Overeaters Anonymous.* Rio Rancho, NM: Overeaters Anonymous, Inc.

Food Addicts in Recovery Anonymous. (2015). *Food Addicts in Recovery Anonymous.* Woburn, MA: Food Addicts in Recovery Anonymous, Inc.

Brownell and Gold (Eds.) (2012). *Food and Addiction: A Comprehensive Manual.* Chapter 53, Werdell, Philip, "From the Front Lines: A Clinical Approach to Food Addiction." New York: Oxford University Press.

174 National Center on Addiction and Substance Abuse (CASA), Understanding and Addressing Food Addiction: A Science-Based Approach to Policy, Practice and Research. CASA, February, 2016.

175 Werdell, P. (forthcoming 2022). Outcome Research on the

Treatment of Food Addiction. Sarasota, FL: Evergreen.

176 OA, FA and GSA literature

Ifland, J. (2003). *Sugars and Flours: How They Make Us Crazy, Sick and Fat and What to do about It.* 1st Books Library. www.1stbooks.com.

Sheppard, K. (2000). *From the First Bite: A Complete Guide to Recovery from Food Addiction.* Deerfield Beach, FL: Health Communications Inc.

Glenbeigh Psychiatric Hospital of Tampa. (1994). *Patient Handbook.* Tampa, FL: Glenbeigh Hospital.

Foushi, et al., *Food Addiction Recovery, a New Professional Model –the ACORN Primary Intensive.* Available on Amazon..

McCarty, T. (2012). *Shades of Hope: How to Treat Your Addiction to Food.* New York: Berkley Books

Tarman, V. and Werdell, P. *Food Junkies: The truth About food addiction.* Toronto: Dundurn. Available on Amazon.

177 Overeaters Anonymous, www.overeatersanonymous.org

Compulsive Eaters Anonymous—HOW, www.ceahow.org

Food Addicts Anonymous, www.foodaddictsanonymous.org

GreySheeters Anonymous, www.greysheet.org

Food Addicts in Recovery Anonymous, www.foodaddicts.org

Overcomers Outreach, www.overcomersoutreach.org

Overeaters Anonymous—HOW, www.oahow.org

Overeaters Anonymous 90-Day Meetings, www.oasv.org/html/90day.htm

Recovery from food Addiction, Inc., www.recoveryfromfoodaddiction.org

See also: "A Tool Kit for Food Addiction Assessment and Treatment; the Basics from A to Z, for Physicians, Dietitians, Therapists and Other Allied Health Professionals." Available at umassmed.edu/psychiatry/

Trimpey, J. (1996). *Rational Recovery: The New Cure for Substance Addiction*. New York: Pocket Books, Simon & Schuster Inc.

Thompson, S. (2017). *Bright Line Eating: The Science of Living Happy, Thin, and Free*. New York: Hay House, Inc.

Beck, J. (2008). *The Beck Diet Solution: Train Your Brain to Think Like a Thin Person*. Birmingham, AL: Oxmoor House.

Heller, R. and Heller, R.F. (1991). *The Carbohydrate Addict's Diet: The Lifelong Solution to Yo-Yo Dieting*. New York: Dutton, Division of Penguin Books.

Roth, G. (2010). *Women, Food and God: An Unexpected Path to Almost Everything*. NY: Scribner.

Barnard, N. (2003). *Breaking the Food Seduction: The Hidden Reasons behind Food Cravings—and 7 Steps to End Them Naturally*. New York: St. Martin's Press.

178 Werdell, P. (2009). Bariatric Surgery and Food Addiction: Preoperative Considerations. Sarasota, FL: Evergreen Press.

179 Warren, R. et al. (2013). The Daniel Plan: 40 Days to a Healthier Life. Published by The Daniel Plan. Also available as a Zondervan Ebook at www.zondervan.com/ebooks

180 Sanders-Butler, Y. (2005). Healthy Kids, Smart Kids. NYC: Penguin Group.

181 Minirth, F. et al. (1991). Love Hunger: Recovery from Food Addition-10-Stage Life Plan for Your Body, Mind, and Soul. New York: Random House.

Spero, D. (2006). *Diabetes: Sugar-Coated Crisis*. Canada: New Society Publishers.

Ifland, J., et al. "Refined food addiction: A classic substance use disorder." *Medical Hypotheses,* www.elsevier.com/locate/mehy

182 Many people just attend these groups as "diet support" without doing the full Twelve Step program. In early-stage food addiction, this is often sufficient for Detox and maintenance of a simple physical abstinence. FA report a bariatric surgeon who requires patients to attend FA before and after the operation. GDA is usually for food addicts whose disease has progressed much further, but many attend meetings and work with a sponsor for an entire year just establishing their physical program; there are short phone meetings three times a day for those needing a lot of support.

183 Overeaters Anonymous. (1980). Overeaters Anonymous, Vol. I. Rio Rancho, NM: Overeaters Anonymous, Inc.

Overeaters Anonymous. (2001). *Overeaters Anonymous, Vol. II.* Rio Rancho, NM: Overeaters Anonymous, Inc.

184 They eliminate sugar, flour, and other binge foods; they use a nutritionally balanced food plan with three meals a day, nothing in between.

185 OA How, OA 90 Days eliminates sugar, flour, and other binge foods; they use a nutritionally balanced food plan with three meals a day, nothing in between, oa.org.

186 Appleton, N. (2009). Suicide by Sugar: A Startling Look at Our #1 National Addiction. Garden City Park, NY: Square One Publishers.

187 Schaub, E. (2014). Year of No Sugar. Naperville, Illinois: Sourcebook.

188 Prager, M. (2010). Fat Boy, Thin Man, Amazon.com

189 Bullitt-Jonas, M. (1998). Holy Hunger: A Woman's Journey from Food Addiction to Spiritual Fulfillment. New York: Vintage.

190 White Bison. (2002). The Red Road to Wellbriety in the Native American Way. Colorado Springs, Colorado: White Bison Inc.

There is a more specific focus on food addiction in their article calling for native people to discard the cultural food ritual of eating friend bread.

191 Norstrand, B. (2019). Living with the Enemy: An Explorations of Addiction and Recovery. Beavers Pond Press.

192 Danowski, D. (2002). Locked Up for Eating Too Much: The Diary of a Food Addict in Rehab. Center City, MN: Hazelden, 2002.

193 Denizet-Lewis, Benoit, America Anonymous: Eight Addicts in Search of a Life. New York: Simon & Schuster, 2009.

194 Ifland, J., et al., "Refined food addiction: A classic substance use disorder." Medical Hypotheses, www.elsevier.com/locate/mehy

195 Pam from Auburn MA. (2004). Sweet Surrender: Christian 12-Step Recovery from Food Addiction. Available on Amazon.

196 Batarseh, Raja, My Yellow Suit: A Lifelong Quest to Lose Weight and Gain Happiness. www.myyellowsuit.com/raja@myyellowsuit.com

197 Brownell, K. and Gold, M. (2012). Food and Addiction: A Comprehensive Handbook, New York: Oxford University Press.

Taubes, G. (2017). *The Case Against Sugar.* New York: Knopf Doubleday Publishing Group. Also:

Sifferlin, A. "Artificial Sweeteners Are Linked to Weight Gain—Not Weight Loss." Source: 7/17/2017 article available at www.Time.com/4859012/artificial-sweeteners-weight-loss/

Brownell, K. and Gold, M. (2012). *Food and Addiction: A Comprehensive Handbook,* New York: Oxford University Press also provides updated corroborating research.

Hyman, M. (2018). *Food: What the Heck Should I Eat?* New York: Little-Brown.

198 Physicians

Dr. Vera Tarman, *Food Junkies: The Truth about Food Addiction.*

Toronto: Dundurn, 2014.

Dr. Neal Barnard, *Breaking the food Seduction.* New York: St. Martin's Press, 2003.

Dr. Beth Rocchio, *Food Addition Treatment: Nature, Assessment and Principles of Treatment* and *Treating Food Addiction, Book 1: The Basics,* available on Amazon.com.

Dr. Philip Kavanaugh, *Magnificent Addiction: Discovering Addiction as Gateway to Healing.* Asian Publishing, 1992.

Dr. Gerald May, *Addiction and Grace.* San Francisco: Harper San Francisco, Division of Harper Collins, 1991.

Dr. Abraham Twerski, *Addictive Thinking: Understanding Self-Deception.* Center City, MN: Hazelden, 1997.

Dr. Pamela Peeke, *The Hunger Fix: The Three-Stage Detox and Recovery Plan for Overeaters and Food Addiction.* NY: Rodale, 2012.

Bariatric Surgery

Mitchell, James E., and Martina de Zwaan, *Bariatric Surgery: A Guide for Mental Health Professionals.* New York: Routledge, 2005.

Werdell, Philip, *Bariatric Surgery and Food Addiction: Preoperative Considerations.* Sarasota, FL: Evergreen, 2009. Also available on Amazon.com.

Stapleton, Connie PhD, *Weight Loss Surgery Does Not Treat Food Addiction.* Mind Body Health Services Inc., 2017.

Therapists

Epstein, Dr. Rhona, *Food Triggers: End Your Craving: Eat Well and Live Better.* Brentwood, TN: Worthy Publishing, 2013.

Katherine, A. (1996). *Anatomy of a Food Addiction: Brain Chemistry of Overeating.* Carlsbad, CA: Gurze Books.

Hollis, J. (1985). *Fat is a Family Affair.* Center City, MN: Hazelden.

Sheppard, K. (2000). *From the First Bite: A Complete Guide to*

Recovery from Food Addiction. Deerfield Beach, FL: Health Communications Inc.

Ifland, J. (2003). *Sugars and Flours: How They Make Us Crazy, Sick and Fat and What to Do about It*. 1st Books Library, www.1stbooks.com.

Kline, M. (19183). *The Junk Food Withdrawal Manual*. Denver, CO: Nutri-Books Corp.

Werdell, P., Foushi, M., Weldon, C. (2007). *The ACORN Primary Intensive: A New Model of Professional Support for Food Addiction Recovery*. Sarasota, FL: Evergreen. Available on Amazon..

199 https://www.ncbi.nlm.nih.gov/pmc/articles/PMC3913362/

200 Beyond Our Wildest Dreams: The Story of the Fellowship of Overeaters Anonymous

201 Overeaters Anonymous, Abstinence. Rio Rancho, NM: Overeaters Anonymous, Inc.

Overeaters Anonymous. (2010). *Dignity of Choice*. Rio Rancho, NM: Overeaters Anonymous, Inc.

202 Overeaters Anonymous (2018). The Twelve Steps and Twelve Traditions of Overeaters Anonymous. Rio Rancho, NM: Overeaters Anonymous, Inc.

203 Wolborsky, B. (1981). "A Survey of Overeaters Anonymous Groups and Membership in North America." Rio Rancho, NM: Overeaters Anonymous, Inc.

204 Bulimics Anonymous, Eating Disorders Anonymous, Anorexics and Bulimics Anonymous: http://aba12steps.org/

205 Overcomers Outreach, https://www.overcomersoutreach.org/

206 Thompson, S. (2017). Bright Line Eating: The Science of Living Happy, Thin, and Free. New York: Hay House, Inc.

Also: Warren, R. et al. (2-13). *The Daniel Plan: 40 Days to a Healthier Life*. Published by The Daniel Plan. Also available as a

Zondervan Ebook at www.zondervan.com/ebooks

Trimpey, J. (1996). *Rational Recovery: The New Cure for Substance Addiction*. New York: Picket Books, Division of Simon & Schuster Inc.

207 Wolborsky, B. (1981). "A Survey of Overeaters Anonymous Groups and Membership in North America." Rio Rancho, NM: Overeaters Anonymous, Inc.

208 "Gallup Survey of Overeaters Anonymous Members." Rio Rancho, NM: Overeaters Anonymous, Inc., 1992.

209 "Overeaters Anonymous Membership Survey." Rio Rancho, NM: Overeaters Anonymous, Inc., 2002.

210 "Overeaters Anonymous Membership Survey," Rio Rancho, NM: Overeaters Anonymous, Inc., 2010.

211 "Overeaters Anonymous Membership Survey," Rio Rancho, NM: Overeaters anonymous, Inc., 2017.

212 Werdell, P. (Forthcoming 2022). Outcome Research on the Treatment of Food Addiction. Sarasota, FL.

213 Kriz, K. (2002). "The Efficacy of Overeaters Anonymous in Fostering Abstinence in Binge-Eating Disorder and Bulimia Nervosa," Virginia Polytechnic Institute, Falls Church, VA.

214 2011 FA Membership Survey

215 2016 FA Membership Survey

216 The name of this organization has been changed from ACORN Food Dependency Recovery Services to SHiFT--Recovery by Acorn.

217 Olofdotter, O. A. (2017). "Survey of MFM Outcome." MFM Reykjavik, Iceland.

218 Ibid.

219 Foushi, M., Weldon, C., and Werdell, P. (2007). The ACORN

Primary Intensive: A New Model of Professional Support for Food Addiction Recovery. Sarasota, FL: Evergreen. Available on Amazon..

220 89% women, 11% men. Almost all were middle and upper income. 89% Caucasian, 11% minorities. 81% consulted a doctor, dietician or counselor about weight, eating or food problems. 70% reported prior therapy for trauma from physical, emotional and/or sexual abuse. 81% reported blood relative with food or alcohol abuse problems. 91% tried three or more diets; 59% tried ten or more. Most had prior experience in a food-related Twelve Step program. 75% had spent more than $5000 on therapy; 19% had spent more than $50,000 out of pocket.

221 Hillock, C., Prager, M. and Werdell, P. "Research Outcomes on ACORN Events." Presented in 2009 at the First National Conference on Promising Practices in Food Addiction Treatment in Houston TX sponsored by the Refined Food Addiction Foundation Research Foundation.

222 Fifteen hundred active alumnae were sent questionnaires; 256 responded. The group had similar characteristics to the general ACORN population.

223 Carroll, Mary Theodora, "The Eating Disorder Inventory and Other Predictors of Successful Symptom Management in Bulimic and Obese Women Following an Inpatient Treatment Program Employing an Addictions Paradigm." A dissertation submitted in partial fulfillment of the requirements for the degree of Doctor of Philosophy in Curriculum and Instruction with an Emphasis in Counselor Education in the Department of Psychological and Social Foundations in the University of South Florida, April, 1993.

224 Pretlow, R. A. (2009). Overweight: What Kids Say. What's Really Causing the Childhood Obesity Epidemic? North Charleston, SC: CreateSpace. Also:

Pretlow, R. (2011). "Addiction to Highly Pleasurable Food as a Cause of the Childhood Obesity Epidemic: A Qualitative Internet Study." Eating Disorders: The Journal of Treatment & Prevention,

19:4, 295-307.

225 Sanders-Butler, Y. (2005). Healthy Kids, Smart Kids. New York: Penguin Group.

226 Gold, Mark, Online Conference Presenter on the Science of Food Addiction at the Eating Disorder Hope Online Conference II, 2018.

227 https://www.healthline.com/health-news/why-drinking-problems-develop-after-weight-loss-surgery

228 In-service panel for professionals on transferring from food addiction to other addictions, Glenbeigh Psychiatric Hospital of Tampa, 1994.

229 Tarman, V. (2014). Food Junkies: The Truth about Food Addiction. Toronto: Dundurn.

230 Alcoholics Anonymous. (2001). Alcoholics Anonymous. New York: Alcoholics Anonymous World Service, Inc., Fourth Edition.

231 These are stories from residential treatment for late and final stage food addiction at Glenbeigh Psychiatric Hospital of Tampa between 1988 and 1996. In the monthly lecture on social consequences of food addiction, each month Werdell asked the therapeutic community of self-assessed food addicts if they personally had experiences of auto accidents or near accidents while eating out of control. there was no formal research on the matter, but about half of the attendees raised their hands each month.

232 https://www.washingtonpost.com/news/to-your-health/wp/2015/06/29/sugary-drinks-linked-to-180000-deaths-a-year-study-says/?noredirect=on

233 https://www.drugabuse.gov/related-topics/trends-statistics/overdose-death-rates

https://opioids.thetruth.com/o/the-facts/fact-1005

https://www.wvdhhr.org/bph/oehp/obesity/mortality.htm

In 2017, there were 47,600 opioid deaths; in 2018, there were 70,137 deaths from all drugs. The annual death rate for obesity is 280,184; and if 1/3 of the obese are food addicted—a modest estimate—then over 90,000 deaths per year are caused by food addiction.

234 Overeaters Anonymous. (2018). Twelve Steps and Twelve Traditions of Overeaters Anonymous. Rio Rancho, NM: Overeaters Anonymous, Inc., pp. 9-11.

235 Milkman, H. and Sunderwirth, G. (1987). Craving for Ecstasy: The Consciousness and Chemistry of Escape. Lanham, MD: Lexington Books. Obese men have a higher incidence of cancer, including colon, rectum and prostate. Overweight women are at a greater risk for developing malignant tumors of the ovaries, uterine lining and, after menopause, of the breasts.

236 Appleton, N. (1996). Lick the Sugar Habit. New York: Penguin Putnam, 1996.

237 Ibid.

238 https://www.nih.gov/news-events/news-releases/nih-study-finds-extreme-obesity-may-shorten-life-expectancy-14-years

239 Cawley J and Meyerhoefer C. "The Medical Care Costs of Obesity: An Instrumental Variables Approach." Journal of Health Economics, 31(1): 219-230, 2012; also:

Finkelstein, Trogdon, Cohen, et al. (2009). "Annual Medical Spending Attributable to Obesity." Health Affairs.

240 www.foodaddictioninstitute.org

241 Cawley, Ibid.

242 https://www.stateofobesity.org/healthcare-costs-obesity/

243 Cawley J., Rizzo JA, Haas K. "Occupation-Specific Absenteeism Costs Associated with Obesity and Morbid Obesity." Journal of Occupational and Environmental Medicine, 49(12):1317-24, 2007.

244 Gates D., Succop P., Brehm B., et al., "Obesity and Presenteeism: The Impact of Body Mass Index on Workplace Productivity." J Occ Envir Med, 50(1):39-45, 2008.

245 Finkelstein EA, Trogdon JG, Cohen JW, Dietz W. "Annual Medical Spending Attributable to Obesity: Payer- and Service-Specific Estimates." Health Affairs, 28(5): w822-831, 2009.

246 The Robert Wood Johnson Foundation, the American Stroke Association, and the American Heart Association. (2005). A Nation at Risk: Obesity in the United States, A Statistical Sourcebook. Callas, TX: American Heart Association.

247 Trust for America's Health. (2008). Prevention for a Healthier America: Investments n Disease Prevention Yield Significant Savings, Stronger Communities. Washington, DC: Trust for America's Health.

248 https://obesitynewstoday.com/reasons-for-not-losing-weight-after-bariatric-surgery/

   Also: Stapleton, C. (2017). *Weight Loss Surgery Does Not Treat Food Addiction.* Mind Body Health Services Inc.

249 Werdell, P. (2009). Bariatric Surgery & Food Addiction: Preoperative Considerations. Sarasota, FL: EverGreen Publications. Also available on Amazon.com.

250 Testimony by Norma at the 2nd Annual Conference on Food Addiction and Bariatric Surgery sponsored by the University of Massachusetts School of Psychiatry and the Food Addiction Institute, October 15, 2015.

251 Clinical observations at a series of ACORN Food Dependency Recovery Primary Intensives, 2011-2013.

252 Testimony by Summer at the 2nd Annual Conference on Food Addiction and Bariatric Surgery sponsored by the University of Massachusetts School of Psychiatry and the Food Addiction Institute, October 15, 2015.

253 Unpublished research by Dr. Douglas Ziedonis, et al., at Bariatric Surgery Program of UMass Medical Center, Memorial Campus, Worcester, MA.

254 Sandoiu, A. "Weight Loss Surgery May Cause Alcohol Addiction," published in Surgery for Obesity and Related Diseases, May 22, 2017.

255 Food Addicts in Recovery Anonymous (2015). Food Addicts in Recovery Anonymous. Woburn, MA: Food Addicts in Recovery Anonymous, Inc., pp. 12=13; www.foodaddicts.org

256 Clinical observations at a series of ACORN Food Dependency Recovery Primary Intensives, 2014.

257 Werdell, P. (2009). Bariatric Surgery & Food Addiction: Preoperative Considerations. Sarasota, FL: EverGreen Publications. Also available on Amazon.com.

258 Werdell, P. (2009). Bariatric Surgery & Food Addiction: Preoperative Considerations. Sarasota, FL: EverGreen Publications. Also available on Amazon.com.

259 Food addiction powerlessness does not mean that food addicts are always unable to stop. It is more complex than this and more difficult. There are times when food addicts can pull back from cravings and will not have mental obsessions about food. Powerlessness over food means that food addicts do not know whether or not they will be able to be in control.

260 In Twelve Step literature, addictive personality is often called "extreme self-centeredness" or "self-will run riot." Alcoholics Anonymous, Alcoholics Anonymous. New York: Alcoholics Anonymous World Service, Inc., Fourth Edition, 2001.

261 Werdell, P. (2012). Food Plans for Food Addiction Recovery, Sarasota, FL: Evergreen. In Chapter 2, we discuss that food abstinence is sometimes more complicated than abstinence in alcoholism and drug addiction. As Dr. Lutzig points out, abstinence from specific foods is dependent upon "Intensity and duration." See:

262 Lustig, R. (2013). *Fat Chance: Beating the Odds Against Sugar, Processed Food, Obesity and Disease.* New York, NY: Hudson St Press.

263 Werdell, P. (2010). Inventorying food slips: Physically, Emotionally, Mentally and Spiritually. Sarasota, FL: Evergreen. Available on Amazon..

264 Definition of abstinence by American Association of Addiction Medicine (ASAM), American Society of Addiction Medicine (ASAM), "Definition of Addiction," https://www.asam.org/resources/definition-of-addiction

265 Twerski, A. (1997). Addictive Thinking: Understanding Self-Deception. Center City, MN: Hazelden.

266 The concept of a blank spot is the language used in Twelve Step programs. Alcoholics Anonymous. (2001). Alcoholics Anonymous. New York: Alcoholics Anonymous World Service, Inc., Fourth Edition. From a clinical point of view, a blank spot is a very small blackout, i.e., the memory being completely blank or blacked out at a particular time.

267 This is a typical example of what it means to say that addiction is "a disease of forgetting."

268 Such an attitude is not unusual in late-stage alcoholics and drug addicts, but the general public and health professionals often are themselves blind to the fact that food addicts also get to this stage.

269 Nakken, C. (1996). The Addictive Personality: Understanding the Addictive Process and Compulsive Behavior. Center City, MN: Hazelden.

270 Twerski, A. (1997). Addictive Thinking: Understanding Self-Deception. Center City, MN: Hazelden.

271 Alcoholics Anonymous. (2001). Alcoholics Anonymous. New York: Alcoholics Anonymous World Service, Inc., Fourth Edition.

272 Tarman, V. (2014). Food Junkies: The Truth about Food Addiction. Toronto: Dundurn.

273 Wilson, G.T., in Fairburn and Wilson (Eds) (1993). Binge Eating: Nature, Assessment and Treatment. New York: Guilford Press. (Wilson cites the work of Bemis, "Phobia, Obsession or Addiction: What Underlies Eating Disorders?" a paper presented at the National Conference on Eating Disorders, Columbus, Ohio, 1985; Rodin and Reed, "Sweetness and Eating Disorders," in Dobbing (Ed) Sweetness; Springer-Veriag, and Wardle, "Compulsive Eating and Dietary Restraints," British Journal of Clinical Psychology, 1987).

Peele, S. (2009). *Diseasing of America: Addiction Treatment Out of Control.* Boston, MA: Houghton-Mifflin.

274 Cheren, M., et al. (2009). Physical Craving and Food Addiction, Food Addiction Institute, www.foodaddictioninstitute.org

American Psychiatric Association, *Diagnostic and Statistical Manual of Mental Disorders Fifth Edition (DSM-5).* Washington, DC: American Psychiatric Publishing, 2013, p. 329.

Note: See more in-depth discussion of the science in Chapter 1 of this book.

275 In Twelve Step programs, this is done by working spiritually on the "First Step." See: Lawrie C. (2016). OA Big Book Study Guide for Compulsive Overeaters. Self-published in Middleton, Delaware, October 18, 2016.

In professional food addiction treatment programs, participants pursue this by writing an in-depth story of the history of their powerlessness over food. See:

Foushi, M., Weldon, C., and Werdell, P. (2007). *The ACORN Primary Intensive: A New Model of Professional Support for Food Addiction Recovery.* Sarasota, FL: Evergreen. Available on Amazon..

276 The name of this organization has been changed from ACORN Food Dependency Recovery Services to SHiFT--Recovery by Acorn.

277 We use the word "spiritual" in a non-religious sense.